To The ...
May yo...
BE Blessed!

Erin's Gift

Never Drive Faster than
your Guardian Angel can Fly

LUKE T. LAWRENCE

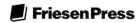

Suite 300 – 852 Fort Street
Victoria, BC, Canada V8W 1H8
www.friesenpress.com

Copyright © 2014 by Luke T Lawrence
First Edition — 2014

All rights reserved.

No part of this publication may be reproduced in any form, or by any means, electronic or mechanical, including photocopying, recording, or any information browsing, storage, or retrieval system, without permission in writing from the publisher.

ISBN   .
978-1-4602-5056-3 (Hardcover)
978-1-4602-5057-0 (Paperback)
978-1-4602-5058-7 (eBook)

1. Medical, Pediatrics

Distributed to the trade by The Ingram Book Company

Table of Contents

Part Three:
TOWARDS THE NEW NORMAL

This book is dedicated in memory of my daughter

Erin Lawrence

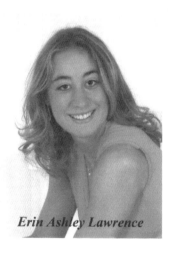

Erin Ashley Lawrence

Foreword

*"Halfway along the path of our life I found myself in a dark forest,
because the straight way had been lost."*
—Dante, The Divine Comedy

I thought my life would be different, my dreams, my hopes, my family, my future. I married the love of my life and had two beautiful children... and then suddenly, the "straight way" was lost. In 1990, my wife RoseMarie was diagnosed with stomach cancer. Seventeen years later my daughter Erin was diagnosed with the same disease. The "disease" was later given a name: Hereditary Diffuse Gastric Cancer. Two months after Erin passed away my son Jared became the youngest person at age eighteen to have his entire stomach surgically removed (Prophylactic Gastrectomy) as a precaution.

I discovered far too late how much my two children had in common with each other and with their mother. Only now am I coming to understand the proverb that a mother's heart is always with her children.

This is our story.

Prologue

Never Drive Faster than your
Guardian Angel can Fly

Like most Saskatchewan winters, it's cold. Damn cold. The year 1991 is only eleven days in and I'm standing ice-fettered among gelid rural memorials close to the western border of Manitoba. She had grown up here, said that she had always loved helping her father with the cattle, taught Sunday school in the town nearby. I feel my two small children sway a touch between sharp blasts of January wind. I move them closer, mooring us slightly deeper in the blowing snow. The three of us might have resembled a baggy anchor, wreathed in tattered sails, half-buried in the sand on some unknown island. We were castaways, our lives a shipwreck.

The wind was still howling when we began the drive back to Regina one week later. Dusting snow clouds rose like ghosts, whirled and swept across the highway in great streaming drifts. The centre line dividing the highway was now completely invisible. It wasn't long before the children were asleep, their breaths quieting down to small sighs buried deep into their coats.

My solitude was absolute. All I could see was a few feet of black pavement in front of me. Everything else was white noise. It was as if I was suspended in some negative space in which there were no pathways, no more signposts to mark the road I was to travel. I wondered whether it would be like this from now on, with only the three of us. I glanced into the rearview mirror. They looked so peaceful, far too young to comprehend what had happened. But whether they comprehended or not, it was certain that their lives had forever changed.

I turned the radio on because I needed something other than the wind and these thoughts. More white noise as the transistors crackle to life. I pushed through the dial, searching for the fragment of a signal, something able to struggle its way through the squall. A song cut through.

Driving home, with the future blank behind a curtain of snow, I noticed something different about every damn love song. Now the lyrics brought up a great swell of memories. My hands began to shake as I fought storms raging both outside and within. I thought that I caught the sound of the wind picking up again, but it could have been the children, breathing small.

Just east of a town called Grenfell, I glance into my rearview mirror and notice the distinctive outline of an RCMP cruiser pulling a u-turn and begin flashing its lights, the red and blue strobes dim through blown snow. I pull over, turn the radio off and began rolling down the window, catching a buckshot of frozen wind, cooling the salt-warm tears streaking my face.

"Do you realize how fast you were going?"

"No, uh no I didn't, officer."

"Where are you coming from today, sir?"

I didn't answer, so he said "Sir?" again, this time a little more insistently. What do you say? What can you say?

The officer whipped out a small leather-bound booklet and a pen, which he gave two shakes to loosen the freezing ink, and began writing.

I didn't know quite how to say it, so I simply said it, all of it. It was the only thing that I could say.

"We buried their mother, my wife, in Rocanville last week. Cancer."

The officer's pen stopped in mid-stroke. I think it was then that he noticed my eyes, bloodshot dry from crying. I watched as he caught sight of the children still asleep, buckled tightly in the back seat and breathing softly through their parkas, warm heaps of small innocence. For a moment things became very still, even the wind seemed to settle. I could hear the breaths between us.

"Have a good day then, sir."

'Have a good day.' I have to admit, it was an odd thing to hear. I admit that I didn't quite know how to take it. It took a minute or two before I realized he hadn't given me a ticket.

A "good day." Thank you.

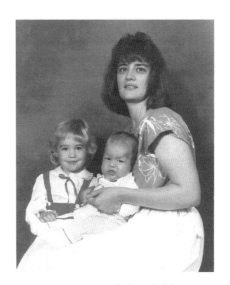

RoseMarie and the Children

Part I
ROSEMARIE

Chapter One

ROSEMARIE

"Whoever said winning isn't everything,
never had to fight CANCER."
—*Unknown*

My son Jared Ryan Lawrence was born on April 25, 1989. In the first eleven months of his life, students protested in Tiananmen Square, the SkyDome opened in Toronto, the Berlin Wall fell, the first McDonald's opened in Moscow, Nelson Mandela was freed after twenty-seven years in prison, and Jared's mom, my wife, RoseMarie began to feel a strangely intense pain in her stomach. The world was becoming a very different place. My world was about to become a very different place. But I wasn't really thinking about that as I drove my wife to the Emergency Room at the Pasqua Hospital in Regina, Saskatchewan.

March 1990

After a brief stint in the Emergency Room, RoseMarie was admitted to the Gastrointestinal (GI Unit.) She was booked to have a "gastroscopy" under the supervision of a specialist by the name of Dr. McHattie. In medical terms, a gastroscopy or "esophagogastroduodenoscopy," is a "diagnostic endoscopic" procedure, which involves looking "inside" the body (Greek: *endo* = within), usually by inserting a snake-like rubber scope with a small camera and light attached down the esophagus. The camera allows the doctors to see into the upper part of the gastrointestinal tract without requiring any incisions into the major body cavities.

After the exam, Dr. McHattie delivered an unexpected blow: they had found cancer in RoseMarie's stomach. Things began happening very quickly. RoseMarie was admitted into the hospital by our family doctor, Dr. McMillan, and immediately referred to see a surgeon by the name of Dr. Hubbard. Pathology reports would later indicate that the disease had gone undetected and had been masked by RoseMarie's pregnancy. The vomiting and acute abdominal pain we thought were symptoms of pregnancy was in fact the first kicking of the disease. Signs we thought meant life were in reality auguries of death.

Dr. Hubbard told us that *"for strong cancer you needed strong medicine,"* intimating that RoseMarie would probably need chemotherapy after surgery. A day later, the doctors read the results of the pathology report and recommended that RoseMarie undergo a gastrectomy, a partial or full surgical removal of the stomach. This was something that I had never heard of or had even imagined was possible. It had to be an awful feeling knowing that when you awoke from surgery you would only have part of your stomach, or no stomach at all. I suppose it was better than the alternative – the disease.

March 16th – RoseMarie and I sat nervously in a hospital room, waiting for the porter to take her to surgery. It was around 1:30 in the afternoon when he arrived. I remember the sun streaming between the heavy slats of the hospital blinds, throwing angular shadows across the room, half obscuring the space between us. RoseMarie went into the bathroom, took off her glasses and reminded me with a smile, as if I didn't already know, that she was practically blind without them. When we were dating she had told me that without her glasses, all she could see were shadows. I kept thinking that surgery would be frightening enough on its own: it must have been terrifying to be unable to see anything but shadows.

RoseMarie handed me her wristwatch and said something that I will never forget. *"If something were to happen to me and I die; I want you to carry on without me. You are still young and I would want you to meet someone and love again."* But RoseMarie's words struck me as unbearable to even think about. I tried to still the quiver I felt in my voice and told her that she would be all right, that I would see her on the flip side. The porters swathed in white, stood waiting in the doorway. I watched as they wheeled RoseMarie down the hall and into the elevator. As the chrome doors slid shut, I told her that I loved her.

A nurse told me that the surgery would take at least four hours and that it would be best if I went home. Somebody would call when she was in the Recovery Room. So I drove home, and I waited. RoseMarie's mother Margaret, her sisters Cindy and Melodie, and I sat in the living room for what seemed like forever. Clock ticks marked out some imperceptible time slower than seconds.

Around 4:30 p.m., the phone rang. It was Dr. Hubbard. He said that RoseMarie was now in recovery and should be down in her room around 6:00 p.m. that evening. Then he said that even though they removed two-thirds of her stomach, they couldn't get all of the cancer.

"For every cancer cell we could find under the microscope", he said, "there were four more we couldn't see."

The technical term for this is "Carcinoma of the stomach with Peritoneal Metastasis." Dr. Hubbard referred to it as "Salt & Pepper Cancer" because it looked as though someone had thrown a handful of salt and pepper into RoseMarie's stomach. There were no large tumours; instead, there was a dispersion of malign "seeds" that had spread throughout the wall of RoseMarie's stomach lining and into her abdomen. The full medical term for this type of cancer is "Diffuse Adenocarcinoma" of the stomach. In most cases involving this form of cancer the disease spreads before it could even be detected. As Dr. Hubbard delivered the news, I felt my mind racing, thoughts and emotions confused, scrambling over one another as though the bellwether that held them to their normal places was somehow lost.

Oh my God!... She's only 28... Please God... Our children... Why God?... Why us?

Later that evening I went to visit RoseMarie. I remember waiting for her to return from the Recovery Room and asking myself how I was going to tell my young wife that they didn't get all of the cancer and that it had spread into her abdomen. I could not, would not, lie to her. But I didn't want to tell her the truth. I wanted her to get through just tonight without knowing. I wanted to prevent my emotions from exposing the truth. But when RoseMarie finally opened her eyes and looked at me, she saw through it all.

"They didn't get it all, did they?" Her voice sounded like dry paper.

My mouth went thin and hard. *"No."*

We spent the rest of the evening holding each other, crying and praying together. It was the first time we had ever prayed together and it was the first time we had prayed out loud. The next day, the nurses had RoseMarie out of bed and walking. Involuntarily, RoseMarie's body lurched forward and she grasped onto an IV pole for support. Body curled like an 'S', I could see that RoseMarie was trembling with pain. I saw her face screwed up into a dolorous grimace as she lurched along, step by aching step. I felt utterly helpless. All I could do was watch.

After twelve days in the hospital, RoseMarie was discharged. She was in less discomfort now and was beginning to walk easier. The surgery was over and we now had to prepare for chemotherapy. I had heard of it before but never really knew what to expect. Five days later the Allan Blair Cancer Centre at the Pasqua Hospital called and told us that we had an appointment to see an oncologist.

April 1990

The snow was just about gone when we walked into the Allan Blair Centre for the first time. The place was jammed with people that I assumed were all waiting to see an oncologist. It seemed as though we were the youngest couple that day at the Clinic. They took us into a private room and asked us about family history and whether there was any history of cancer in the family. Well, I don't think I knew anyone who hasn't got a friend or relative that has or had passed away from cancer.

After talking to the doctor, we were informed that the type of gastric cancer from which RoseMarie suffered was both very rare, affecting only one per cent of the world population and, as a result, very difficult to treat. We contacted the Mayo Clinic in Rochester, Minnesota but the initial news wasn't very encouraging. They told us that there was no effective treatment program outside of chemo. The most common chemo drug used for cancer of the stomach is 5Fluorouracil or 5FU, a colorless liquid usually administered through an intravenous line in the back of the hand or in the crook of the arm. The Mayo Clinic recommended that we supplement the use of 5FU with a combination of experimental drugs. This would be considered an "aggressive" approach.

We hoped that adding the experimental drugs would somehow slow down the disease and, with a wing and a prayer, force it into remission. After signing a lot of papers and consents, RoseMarie was put on a program for advanced gastric protocol at the North Central Cancer Treatment Group (NCCTG), a "Chemotherapy research program" based in Rochester consisting of a network of cancer specialists at clinics, hospitals, and medical centers around Canada and the U.S.

April 20th – After having blood drawn and an Electrocardiogram Graph (ECG), a test that measures the electrical activity of the heart, RoseMarie was admitted to Ward 2E in the old wing of the Pasqua Hospital to receive her first dose of 5FU. She was discharged the next day and put on a five-week treatment schedule, which included an injection of "Triazinate" on Day 36. Triazinate is the heavy hitter: this is the chemo drug that kills the cells that are dividing too quickly and becoming cancerous. But here's the rub: Trianzinate doesn't discriminate. It kills every cell it finds, cancerous or not. "Good" cells would be expected to regenerate while the "bad" cells would ultimately die off. It is this process that is the most difficult for the body to sustain. Trianzinate is scorched earth.

May 1990

The whole process was intense. Each time RoseMarie had to be admitted to Ward 2E under observation for a possible drug reaction, each time the drug was administered she had to sign another consent form, and every Monday a follow-up blood test would be required. Between May 22–24, RoseMarie was again admitted to the hospital to begin the second "cycle" of chemo-therapy. She received 375mg of Triazinate through an IV daily for three doses, each dose being added to 500 milliliters of dextrose solution (5%) and infused over one hour. She was also given 25mg of Benadryl to decrease the chance of allergic reactions, and 20mg of metoclopramide to keep her nausea in check.

Just sitting there, waiting for the drugs to run through her system was the most helpless feeling in the world. I just kept taking in the awful thought that the treatment seemed about as bad as the disease. The nurse would come in regularly to check her heart rate and blood pressure. After the drugs were through, we could go home. They gave us a handful of pills for nausea and told her to drink a lot of water, because the chemo would be hard on her kidneys and water would help flush out any concentration of the drugs that could damage them.

On the first day of therapy RoseMarie was vomiting every ten minutes. Gradually, she lost all of her hair and began wearing a wig. RoseMarie was in a great deal of pain, constantly nauseated and vomiting, but she never complained. Although she was often too sick to eat, she would always try to sit at the dinner table with the rest of us. On one particular day, a day I can recall as though it were yesterday, she looked at me, pale as a ghost and thin as a rail, and said she didn't know what was worse, the chemo or the cancer. She said that she couldn't tell anymore what was actually killing her, and that if she had to do it all over again, she would not have had the chemo.

July 1990

RoseMarie continued chemo treatments with follow-ups to the clinic on July 11th and July 16th. On July 23rd she was hospitalized for a day, deferring a cycle of Triazinate. The chemo had so completely decimated her immune system that she contracted chicken pox, for the *second* time in her life.

July 29th – We went to Pasqua Hospital Emergency where RoseMarie was admitted for the next five days with acute abdominal pain, diarrhea and severe vomiting. We still weren't sure if this was symptomatic of the disease or its treatment. All we could tell for sure was that it had been getting worse. This time we were met by another doctor, Dr. McMillan. We told him we had thought the abdominal pain and discomfort was from the chemotherapy. After examining her, Dr. McMillan referred us once more to Dr. Hubbard. Over the following days, RoseMarie was hooked into an IV to keep her hydrated and to control her vomiting. Anything RoseMarie tried to eat came back up.

She had an X-ray, a pelvic ultrasound, and an upper gastrointestinal (GI) series, which confirmed that – on top of everything else – she had a bowel obstruction. Dr. Hubbard consulted us and after discussing the pending bowel obstruction, we had no choice but to concede to having surgery, yet again.

August 1990

August 8th – RoseMarie was to have another operation. This time we *knew* it was the cancer. We had to wait until RoseMarie's condition was more stable before going under the knife. This was going to be her second operation in a little less than one hundred and fifty days. Things were different, however, this time we were aware of the facts and prayed that Dr. Hubbard could remove the obstruction. The risks were high, but RoseMarie really had no choice: it was either the surgery or starving to death. They were going to perform a "Distal gastrectomy and biopsy of peritoneum" and remove approximately 66% of her stomach.

After the surgery, RoseMarie was brought to the Intensive Care Unit (ICU) for recovery. Only immediate family was allowed in the ICU, which meant that only one of us at a time could visit her, and only for a few minutes. We had to put on a full-length canary yellow gown, a gauzy mask, hat, and slippers over our shoes. When I first walked into ICU, I was completely overwhelmed by all the equipment. There was an intricate network of drainage tubes sticking out of RoseMarie's body in almost every direction imaginable. She was in a great deal of pain – her face was puffy, her eyes watery, and she couldn't speak very well.

The children weren't allowed to visit. I don't think RoseMarie would have wanted them to see her like that anyway, and God knows I didn't. The doctors kept her in ICU for three days before they brought her back to a private room on the ward. After the surgery, Dr. Hubbard told me that the disease had spread almost everywhere and that RoseMarie would only feel well for about two weeks before the tumors would re-obstruct her entire small bowel. "She will die from her tumours," he said. I would never have the heart to tell my wife that she was going to die.

August 17th – RoseMarie was discharged from the hospital a week after her surgery. As the days became weeks and the weeks added up to a month, her quality of life began to visibly deteriorate. It became common to hear and see RoseMarie in the bathroom, vomiting every time she tried to eat or drink anything. She began to lose a lot of weight and found it difficult to keep up with the children. Despite all this, she insisted on bathing the kids, cooking meals, and doing housework for as long as she could.

September 1990

September 14th – On our last visit to the Allan Blair Cancer Centre, RoseMarie wasn't doing well. She needed another surgery and Dr. Hubbard's ominous words kept echoing through my brain: "She will die from her tumours." In a final act of desperation we went to see him. We pleaded with him to reconsider and operate again. He examined her and told us both he would not operate a third time; surgery was impossible. We both left in tears, consumed with the feeling of having been abandoned, lost in a wilderness from which we could not escape, simply waiting to die. I was losing my wife, the children were losing their mother, and our future together as a family was going to be taken away.

December 1990

RoseMarie continued to get weaker by the day. She could no longer take anything orally and seemed to be surviving only on love and prayers. She became very weak and was no longer able to walk. We decided to work with what we had left and, after some convincing, she agreed to get a wheelchair. This was something she didn't want to do; it felt like conceding to the disease. We asked RoseMarie's mom Margaret if she would come to Regina, and help us with the daily chores of raising our two young children. This meant that Margaret would be moving in indefinitely, leaving her husband Ray, their young son Adam and the farm outside of Rocanville. RoseMarie had decided to stay at home as much as possible with the children, rather than be hospitalized.

Our daughter, Erin Ashley Lawrence was four years old, and our son Jared had not even celebrated his second birthday.

So RoseMarie volunteered to trial a pilot program for future cancer patients, becoming the first patient to have IV at home so she could spend as much of the time she had left with her young family. She was permitted to take her IV and pain medication out of the hospital. I had to learn how to give morphine injections and practiced by injecting oranges with water. I also had to learn how to calibrate and operate her IV since there were no automatic injections or IV monitors like we have today. Having Margaret living with us and running the household allowed me to concentrate on helping RoseMarie. We were quite the team. Margaret usually put in twelve-hour days with the children and I was able to spend a lot of quality time with RoseMarie.

We carried on day by day and with Christmas steadily approaching, RoseMarie wanted to get going on our shopping. I rigged a portable IV pole, using a 5/8th inch wooden dowel and a hook, which I then taped to the back leg of the wheelchair. Using this homemade contraption we were now able to attach her IV bag to the chair and leave the house. We made our way in and out of all the department stores. It was far from perfect, grinding our way through the snow and the busy throng of late season shoppers, but it was very important to RoseMarie that she do her own Christmas shopping.

I remember one afternoon we were shopping at The Bay and RoseMarie said that she suddenly felt nauseous. I pushed her wheelchair into a clothes rack so she could vomit into a plastic grocery bag without drawing too much attention. Despite everything, at that moment it seemed as though it was RoseMarie who was in control, and the disease was merely along for the ride. RoseMarie's cancer slowed her down but it never stopped her from doing whatever she thought was important. We became thankful for each day.

Every day I was becoming more and more aware that life is a gift and should never be taken for granted.

The hardest thing to accept was the likelihood that RoseMarie would not see our children grow up. One night I awoke to find her looking into Jared's crib. She said, "I wonder what he will be in life. I'm scared it's taking me away from my babies." RoseMarie never dwelled on herself much or complained about the pain she was obviously suffering. That was her character and her strength. I could see where all of RoseMarie's strength had come from. Margaret dropped everything on the farm to come to Regina and help us out with the cooking, laundry, housework, caring for Erin and Jared and even helping to bathe RoseMarie. I don't think I ever got a chance to sit down and thank her properly for her sacrifice.

January 1991

RoseMarie spent a quiet New Years sleeping on the couch. We never rang in the New Year like most but it didn't really matter. Every single day was a new gift, something we always felt thankful for. RoseMarie made it her goal to survive long enough to see the New Year. At the very least, she had gotten her wish.

The last week of her life RoseMarie slept on the couch in our living room with the fireplace burning at all times. I never knew exactly why she had done this. I do know that RoseMarie was reading her Bible most of the time and found it most comfortable being around people and her family. I remember it like it was yesterday. RoseMarie's family was staying at our house all that week. The fifth night of the New Year was clear and cold. RoseMarie fell gravely ill.

The next day I called Dr. McMillan and told him of RoseMarie's condition and he said he would drop by later that evening. It was about 5:30 p.m. when Dr. McMillan made a house call. He told me that RoseMarie was dying. The weather was extremely cold. I always kept a fire burning at night to keep RoseMarie warm and as comfortable as possible. This night felt different, somehow. Things seemed to be very still, very quiet. All you could hear was the snap and roar of the fire and the smell of smoke as it wisped up the chimney.

Ever since I had first learned of the disease my mind was in a perpetual state of agitation and I found it impossible to sleep. That night was no different. I sat in our living room watching her sleep, stoking the fire, trying to keep her warm. I had the rest of my life to sleep. I wanted to share what precious time we had left together. I would sit beside her every one of those last nights and just watch her. She was so peaceful. I couldn't explain it but I had a feeling that the doctor was right. I knew something was really wrong. This was it. This was really the end.

January 6th – I called the farm and spoke to Clint, RoseMarie's brother. I told him that I was getting low on firewood and he said it was no problem for him to bring a load up with him that night. It was cold that week. So damn cold. It was cold enough that the sun reflected itself into mock suns in the frozen sky, casting a halo of ice. The planes at the Regina Airport sounded as if they were taking off from your own backyard. As Clint and I hauled the firewood from the back of his truck, we could hear the snow dryly snapping under our feet. It was so still, like the world was holding its breath, waiting for something to happen.

I remember I stayed awake all night stoking the fire while RoseMarie was asleep on the sofa. As I lay on the floor in front of the fireplace, a feeling came over me that was hard to describe. It was a feeling of hollowness. The room felt like a vacuum. All the sound in the room seemed to be getting sucked up the chimney along with the smoke. It was so cold outside and so warm inside that the fire seemed to be drawing out every last whiff of breathable air.

January 7th – Sometimes you do things because you have to and not because you want to. It was time to have the children leave the house. RoseMarie's life was almost over and I think she would have asked me to ask the children to leave if she could speak. I didn't want the children to remember something I can't forget. I called Erin's Godparents Charlotte and Terry, and asked them to pick up the children and keep them overnight. RoseMarie carried her own cross. RoseMarie's final hours never found her complaining about the pain or cursing her fate.

I remember this so damn well. RoseMarie was lying on the sofa on her back. It was about 5:20 p.m. and all of her family had gathered around her. I thought I could see in her eyes that the end was near. She could hardly speak and her eyes were full of tears. I was holding her hand as she looked in my eyes. Something told me that she was holding on for her children. I told her that if she saw a light and if that light was calling to her, to go to God. I said, "I promise I will raise the children, I promise." She squeezed my hand just once more. The last tears fell from her face, the last breath fell from her lips, and she was gone.

Chapter Two
FIGHTING A LOSING BATTLE

I sat with RoseMarie until the ambulance quietly rolled into our driveway; no flashing lights, no sirens, just the barely audible crunch of the tires over the snow-skiffed driveway, followed by the sound of the doorbell. RoseMarie's father answered the door and two EMS personnel walked in, carrying a stretcher. They pulled a thin white sheet over RoseMarie's body and took her away.

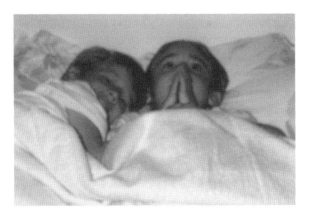

Jared and Erin

On January 8th, I called Charlotte and asked her to bring Erin and Jared home. I didn't know how I was going to tell the children that their mother was gone forever. I was still in shock myself. But I had promised RoseMarie that I would take care of the children and the day after her passing, I knew I had that responsibility. The kids walked through the door with Charlotte and Terry. Everyone was standing in the living room and I could see that Erin was looking for her mother, but she wasn't lying on the sofa anymore.

I hugged them both and tried to explain that "Mommy's gone to heaven and she's not sick any more. We can't see her... but she can see us." Everyone was crying. RoseMarie's father was crushed. I had never seen him cry before. There was this immense pain on his face. The whole scene reminded me of when I lost my father at the age of thirteen, two months after heart surgery. I knew then, and I knew again at that moment, that I would remember this day for the rest of my life.

I had never made funeral arrangements before and didn't even know where to begin. It's just not something I was prepared to think about. My Uncle Don and Aunt Doreen came over the next day and offered their help. We discussed possible arrangements and juggled some ideas around. I finally decided that because our life together had been so brief and because RoseMarie had always told me how much she loved the farm where she had grown up, I would bring her home. I wanted her final resting place somewhere her soul could gaze upon the countryside and there remain a part of the life she left behind. She had always told me about how she loved teaching Sunday school in Rocanville and helping her father with the cattle. We decided that we would have the prayer service in Regina and the funeral service in Rocanville. We contacted Speers Funeral Chapel in Regina and made all the necessary arrangements. A short time later, I met with the chaplain, Father K, to discuss potential readings and hymns. I had requested a special song that was inspirational to me at the time.

Unfortunately, Father K informed that me that the song couldn't possibly be used for the service: the only music allowed at the prayer service would have to come from the *Catholic Book of Worship*. I was disappointed to say the least, but because we had been married in the United Church and had a Catholic priest bless our marriage, I still felt it would be appropriate for there to be a Catholic prayer service in Regina. I was grateful the song could be sang at the funeral in Rocanville.

I hadn't yet decided who I would ask to be RoseMarie's pallbearers. Eventually, I decided on four uncles, two from each side, and two cousins, one from each side. The prayer service was to be held January 10th at St. Peter's Church in Regina. RoseMarie's funeral happened the next day at St. Paul's United Church in Rocanville.

When you check the map, Rocanville doesn't look like much, a two and a half kilometre speck of dust nestled against the provincial border shared by Saskatchewan and Manitoba. The town was briefly thrust onto the international scene when amateur inventor, welder, and machinist Ernie Symons brought his patented oilcan design to town in 1923. One of the first oilcans specifically constructed for use on farm and industrial machinery, Symons' design proved to be the *"best in the world."*

As a result, Rocanville became instrumental in manufacturing thousands of oilcans during World War II to help with the maintenance of aircraft, tanks, and various military impedimenta – a feat since commemorated by a monolithic seventy-foot scale-model of Symons' oiler at the eastern entrance of the town. After the closure of the oilcan factory in the late 1980's, Rocanville is mostly known (if known at all) for its potash mine and livestock farms, which dot the low hills surrounding the town.

RoseMarie's parents farmed livestock, and when I met RoseMarie in the fall of 1982, Symons was still pumping out oil cans. We met at the tail end of what's known to locals as "Agribition" week, which usually happens in around the last two weeks of November. Agribition – a kind of portmanteau of the words Agriculture and Exhibition – is Canada's largest agricultural and livestock fair, and RoseMarie's father was in Regina showing his Black Angus cattle.

Needless to say, a weeklong gathering of farmers and cowboys in the city isn't all business, and almost every night there was some kind of party going on. A friend and I were supposed to meet a couple of girls after one of the Cabarets and eventually make our way to a house party. As I had not yet discovered, the girl I was supposed to get acquainted with wasn't RoseMarie, but her sister, Melodie. After about an hour of milling about and generally having a good time, some girl comes striding through the middle of the party dressed in beat-up coveralls and smelling like a barn. Exchanging slightly embarrassed glances, Melodie introduces her sister, RoseMarie, who began explaining to the bemused partygoers that she had been helping her father with the cattle all day.

I was immediately attracted, not only by her looks, but also by a peculiar mixture of modesty and probity that signalled a kind of inner strength. I thought I sensed something real in her. She didn't seem particularly concerned with trying to impress us and she never pretended to be someone she wasn't. We spent the rest of the evening talking. It was one of those perfect talks where everything else in the world melts away into the background and it's just the two of you. I began to fall in love.

Six months later, I invited RoseMarie to be my escort at my cousin's wedding. Shortly afterwards we began a long distance relationship. RoseMarie still lived on her parents' farm in Rocanville, and I would drive 225 kilometres there and back every weekend. We commuted back and forth between Regina and Rocanville for about two years. I asked RoseMarie to marry me on Valentine's Day, 1983. We were married eighteen months later, on July 14, 1984. I was twenty-three years old.

RoseMarie and I drove along this same stretch of highway many times. This trip was going to be different. I packed enough clothes for the children for a week knowing we wouldn't be home for a while. RoseMarie's service was so emotional, words can't really describe the feeling. I was burying my young wife, only twenty-nine years old, the mother of our babies. Reverend Stevenson had married us in 1984 and it was the same Rev. Stevenson who would oversee RoseMarie's funeral less than seven years later.

After not being able to choose any of the music for the service in Regina, I was so pleased and relieved when Rev. Stevenson agreed to allow *Wind Beneath My Wings* to be sung during the funeral. *Wind* had always been *the Song* for RoseMarie and I. It was sung beautifully by Dawn Wilson, a member of the congregation, and I don't believe anyone could have sung it better; her voice captivated the entire room.

As the song reached its crescendo, RoseMarie's casket began making its way out of St. Paul's United Church and into the winter sun. Rays of light went streaming across the curved face of the casket. I asked the pallbearers to lift her up as high as possible, bringing her as close to God in death as she was in life. In silent prayer, I thought, *RoseMarie did not want to leave this world Lord, but I know now that she is in a better place.* After Rev. Stevenson placed the sign of the cross on RoseMarie's casket, I led the congregation in *The Lord's Prayer*. It was the only prayer we had shared when we were together.

Chapter Three

THE NANNY

*"Life is a classroom in which each of us is being
tested, tried, and passed."*
—Robert Thibodeau

It was only 5:00 p.m. when we finally arrived back home, but it was already dark. I gently woke Erin and carried Jared into the house. I knew the children would be hungry and I quickly put together a makeshift dinner. I planned on feeding Jared first. Erin was already pretty good at feeding herself, but like most two-year-olds, Jared was far more interested in playing with his food than putting it into his mouth.

Erin became a "big" little sister to Jared almost instantly after RoseMarie's death. She was only four at the time and already enjoyed helping Dad out in the kitchen. I was never a big fan of dishwashers and found them to be more of a hassle to load and unload, so we usually did it the old-fashioned way: I would wash and Erin would dry. My hands were always too big to get into the bottom of the glasses, but Erin never had a problem. We became quite the team and sometimes Jared would even join in, drying his own plastic dishes.

Erin and Jared had always enjoyed each other's company. I could see that RoseMarie's absence had the fortunate effect of making the children best friends. She always told me that she would be there for the children, and in these small moments, working together washing and drying our own dishes, I knew that she was.

Soon enough it was February and spring was quickly approaching. I had given a lot of thought to the way things would have to be with RoseMarie gone, and decided on four things:

1. We would stay in our current house and the children would continue going to the same school as they had the year before.

2. I would go back to work as soon as I could, and this meant that...

3. I would need to hire a live-in nanny to care for the children. Finally, as a matter of personal pride, and perhaps a way of working through the shock of losing RoseMarie...

4. I would finish that damn basement.

The first one was easy enough: stay the course. I thought that losing their mother would be hard enough, so at the very least the children would be able to stay in the same neighbourhood and keep all of their friends. The second task, hiring a live-in nanny, would be trickier. I knew as little about hiring nannies as I did about arranging funerals. I would be entrusting my children, the only family I had left, with a complete stranger.

The local phone book sat in front of me, a cold lump, daring me to navigate its deceptively calm waters. I flipped open the Yellow Pages and thumbed to "N." When I got to "Nannies" I found a cross-reference to Immigration Services. After a few phone calls leading nowhere, I eventually got a hold of someone who described themselves as an "agent" responsible for importing nannies from other countries. I wasn't sure if this was legal, but I left a message anyway. Someone called back an hour later and arranged for a meeting at our house.

The agent-man arrived late one evening, accompanied by a woman. We sat in the living room and the man pulled out a large, glossy catalogue, filled with photographs. He began explaining that most of his nannies came from Asia and that they were ready to come to Canada as soon as they were contacted by the agency. I looked over several resumes and noticed that most of the potential nannies were young, attractive, women from the Philippines or Korea between twenty-four and twenty-eight years of age. All of them had some childcare experience in Hong Kong. I decided that I would let Erin make the final decision. She picked and I signed the papers.

The agency required a deposit and informed me that I would have to make an appointment with Immigration, at which point I breathed a sigh of relief; this thing seemed to be legit after all. Immigration let me know that I was required by law to provide our prospective nanny with her own furnished private quarters, including a bathroom, and that I had to pay (at least) minimum wage with Canada Pension Plan benefits. Hours of work would be up to the employer to negotiate and days off had to be scheduled in advance. Our nanny was scheduled to arrive in six to eight weeks. This allowed me to get going on decision number four – the basement.

The outside walls of the basement were already framed and insulated, so I had a bit of a head start. My initial plans were to build private quarters for the nanny, including a large master bedroom with a full three-piece bath. After starting construction, however, I decided to go big casino and finish the whole basement. My neighbour Chris volunteered to help me with some of the framing, painting, and constructing a suspended or *"T-Bar"* ceiling. To speed things up, I decided it would be better if the children visited their grandparents on the farm.

Mom and Dad agreed to keep them for two weeks, leaving me to work all day and most nights on the basement. Chris agreed to come over in the evening and on weekends. We really hauled ass. We had the bedroom completed and the basement completely finished in just two months. It was a good thing too, because our nanny arrived right on schedule, almost eight weeks to the day.

I got Erin and Jared dressed in their Sunday best as we prepared to meet her in the early afternoon. Around 1:00 p.m. the doorbell rang, and a member of the agency escorted our new nanny into the house. She was from the Philippines and in her mid-twenties, wore a red suit, white blouse, and a short skirt with black nylons. Her hair was about shoulder length, jet black. Erin said she had picked her because she was the prettiest, and I couldn't have agreed more.

Our nanny came to us from the Philippines by way of Hong Kong, her Canadian name was "Anna," and she had only one suitcase. Erin liked her right away. She was very pleasant and seemed to take to the children almost immediately. It was a bittersweet feeling to have a strange woman taking care of my children and living with us, but it seemed as though it would be more of an adjustment for me than the children. Erin was going to be five in August and Jared was turning two on the 25th of April. But with a nanny in place, I decided I could now return to work.

The days turned into weeks, and weeks turned into months, and Anna seemed to be working out great. In the thaw of *"muddy May"* we decided to take a trip to the family farm. Since Anna had basically become part of the family, we decided that we would take her along. Having lived much of her life on a small island in the Philippines and in the urban crush of Hong Kong, our nanny couldn't believe all the open space. She couldn't grasp the idea that one person could own so much land and let us know that you couldn't go anywhere in Hong Kong "without people." We were as amazed at her descriptions of Hong Kong's shoulder-to-shoulder population as she was about Canada's wide-open landscapes.

When I first employed our nanny, I had only signed a one-year contract with Immigration. I thought we would likely not be requiring a nanny after Erin began school, so in April of 1992 I began to look for alternative arrangements. Erin was in school all day but Jared, who was only three years old, still needed a babysitter. Over the course of the next year I tried several different sitters but couldn't find anyone that could replace our nanny. I was beginning to think that I had made a big mistake in letting her go.

One morning, the phone rang and it was Jackie Mason, our neighbour two doors down. She said she and her husband had been talking the night before and had decided that they would look after Erin and Jared. I knew she wasn't offering to do this for lack of excitement, since she already had two children. But I did know that they were likely aware of the fact that I was having problems finding a suitable replacement for Anna – hell, I think the whole neighbourhood knew.

Jackie used some lame excuse that made me smile, saying something about how her children got along so well with Erin and Jared and they would be good company for one another. She was practically begging me to consider, and given our situation, I decided that sometimes one can't be so proud as to say "no" to people who are trying to help. I had promised RoseMarie I would take care of the children, so I couldn't say no to Jackie's offer. To this day, Bob and Jackie Mason are two of the nicest people you could ever meet. I had a feeling this was an answer to my prayers.

Chapter Four

NEW RELATIONSHIP

Slowly, but not a little unsurely, things were beginning to fall into place. Erin was now in school and Jared had fantastic sitters in Bob and Jackie. I had been back to work for a few months, now as a Customer Service Technician for the provincial phone company, Sask-Tel. One of my responsibilities was to look after service in what's known as the "South District Route," which includes a chain of small towns south of Regina: Milestone, Wilcox, Rouleau, Avonlea, Riceton, Estlin, and Grey.

I was on one of my runs through Wilcox, a small village about forty minutes south of Regina and home to the Athol Murray College of Notre Dame. Notre Dame is probably best known for its tradition of pumping out quality NHL players: Vincent Lecavalier, Brad Richards, Rod Brind'Amour, Curtis Joseph, Wendel Clark, among others can be found on the "wall of fame" in the foyer of the school's Olympic-sized hockey rink. For me, it's less the impressive hockey tradition than the school's Latin motto that I remember: *Luctor et Emergo* – "Struggle and Emerge" – a phrase that seemed very appropriate for the next big change that was about to occur in my life, and an enduring lesson for the changes I would encounter not too far down the road.

The name of this first big change was Jan. She was training at the college on a new switchboard that a co-worker and I were installing at the time. We were working in the telephone room at the school when I saw a flash of red and a great pair of stems wandering past the half-opened door. We had just completed transferring the school to a new phone system and were in the process of setting up a temporary training facility in the boardroom. The administrators had asked us to make some last minute programming changes for a Superset – a digital phone capable of multiple lines appearing on a single set – that Jan would be using for her training.

When I walked into the room I saw a very tall, very attractive, blonde woman wearing a smart red two-piece suit, white nylons, and a short skirt with high heel shoes. As we installed the Superset, I stole more than a few glances Jan's way. I never thought I would meet her again, nor did I even plan to. But if I've learned anything, I've learned this: never say never, and the answer will always be 'no' unless you ask. It had been about eleven months since RoseMarie had passed away. I hadn't ever considered going out anywhere, with anyone. I was Mr. Mom. I went to work, came home, started supper, and put the kids to bed. Like clockwork. With apologies to Hamlet, the 'time' was about to be knocked 'out of joint,' yet again.

Every now and then the workers' union at Sask-Tel would hold dances for its members. On one particular occasion, I decided to call up Ron Shatkowski, an old buddy of mine from school, to ask if he wanted to go stag. I knew he and his girlfriend had recently split and this would be an ideal time, for both of us, to have a guy's night out. I would supply the tickets if Ron supplied the wheels. It didn't take much arm-twisting and Ron agreed right away. I arranged a sitter for the kids and we struck out into the night like a couple of teenagers.

I'll admit it, I hadn't felt this good in awhile. When we got to the dance Ron seemed to know as many people as I did. We were standing around BS'ing near the bar when the house band began playing a jumpy fast one. A woman approached and said she had a friend that would like to dance with me, but was too shy to ask herself.

I hadn't danced at all since RoseMarie passed away. The thought was strange enough to me that I instinctively thought someone was pulling a prank. I threw a skeptical grin at Ron and followed her through increasingly thick curtains of cigarette smoke to the second floor of the dancehall. The smoke was so thick by the time we reached the landing that I could hardly make anything out. I glimpsed another flash of red, lightning cochineal through the billowing grey pall. The woman's friend stood up: it was Jan. I laughed at the coincidence and led her downstairs to the dance floor without a second thought. It was the beginning of a new relationship.

It wasn't too long before Jan and I began seeing each other. Jan had no children of her own, and I wasn't sure what the situation would be like when I first brought her around to meet Erin and Jared. I wasn't too worried about Jared; he was still in diapers and would probably adapt easily enough. Things could have been trickier with Erin, who was old enough to have clear memories of her mother.

Nevertheless, Erin seemed to accept Jan straight away and this made things easier. There would still be some fine-tuning, however. I remember the first night I brought her over, Jared needed to be changed. I was busy doing something with Erin at the time, so I asked Jan if she might take care of it for me. She cheerfully agreed and disappeared with the diaper bag. Twenty minutes went by and I'm beginning to wonder what's taking so long. As I cross into the next room, Jan leaps up and triumphantly presents a freshly changed Jared. The only problem was that the diaper was on backwards!

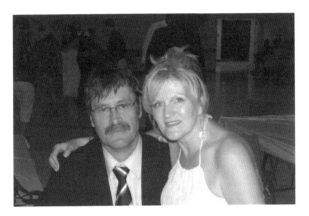

Myself and Jan

At the time I took it for granted that all women knew more about these types of things than men, but as I had already discovered from our experience with the nanny, sometimes what people have most in common is how much they have yet to learn.

Time passed. The kids were getting used to having Jan around and we were becoming more and more of a family. In 1997, we decided to do our first big family trip together. We booked a flight to Orlando, Florida to see – who else? – Mickey Mouse. The children were now eleven and eight, and this would turn out to be the first of four trips to Florida. We planned to be there for three weeks.

As many parents can likely relate, the first big trip to 'the happiest place on earth' with young ones is something of an endurance test. It largely consists of long, incredibly hot, days pounding pavement, seemingly endless queues, absolute proximity to equally sweaty and potentially irritable throngs of tourists, and near complete physical and mental (re: 'It's a Small World') exhaustion. Disney may call itself the happiest place on earth, but it also makes damn sure that you *earn* that happiness. After each day, I imagined I felt that I had conquered a small country – which, in its own way, Disney is.

The first week we decided to stay at one of the Disney Resorts. Jan had already been to Disney World once before, so she served as our tour guide and made sure we hit everything we needed to see in the theme parks and water parks. Already completely exhausted after a week at Disney World, we decided that we would spend the last two weeks of the trip touring the rest of Florida. I rented a car and we made our way through the Sunshine State.

We enjoyed ourselves so much that Jan and I decided to purchase a timeshare for a week every year, thinking it would give us a good excuse to travel. As a result, we were able to make four trips to Florida in the span of eight years, along with two ocean cruises, before Erin began her second year of university.

Throughout the intervening years, Jan and I fell in love. We were about to share a life and a family together. I always have this image of us as if we were *The Brady Bunch*, the perfect TV family, except that Jan was divorced and had no children from her previous marriage. I believed things were happening for a reason, and that maybe Jan and I were meant for each other. Our paths began in different directions and seemed to have met in the middle.

After having lost the 'straight way' on life's path, it seemed as though I had found a thread that would help me find it once more. I tried to be realistic. I looked very closely at our relationship and compared it with other families whose children were raised by both biological parents. All families had personal problems and sometimes never got along. As Erin in particular got older, we wouldn't be any different. I kept telling myself that our family was no different than any other that had two females living under the same roof. My little girl was growing up. Her hair, once the colour of spun gold, was now streaked with a handsome brunette. She was transforming before my eyes from a child into a mature and attractive young woman.

CODA: Letters to RoseMarie

A Mother's Eternal Love

You were taken away from me before I was old enough to realize what it was going to mean to be without you for the rest of my life. I want you to know that I love and miss you more and more each day. There is not one day that you have not passed through my mind. I think about you all the time, and I can promise that I will never forget you.

I want you to know that I do my best everyday in hope as not to let you down. I am trying to live my life in a way that would make you proud. Words cannot express the void that I feel without having you in my life. I know that you and I would get along wonderfully, and that we would understand one another better than anyone else could.

I long so badly to have you here with me through all the moments of my life, and through all of the monumental moments I will be experiencing. Even though I know that you are always close by, and that you watch over me, I cannot help but wish that I still had you here with me. Most of all, I just want to let you know, that you were, are, and always will be my mother, and that I will never forget you in all the days of my life. You are my strength, my role model, and my will.

I love you with all of my heart.

Erin Lawrence

★ ★ ★

A Deadly Disease

A mother with a deadly disease
Has no hope any longer.
She will be gone soon leaving
her family and kids.

Why can't there be more time?
To see them grow up and to
Be with them.

She will be gone soon.

Watching from above,

Keeping them safe with her unconditional love.

Erin Lawrence

★ ★ ★

A Childhood Experience

When growing up through childhood she's the one you can
always count on. The one who is always there for you no
matter what happens. What happens if she's not there? You
know she's there in spirit but not physically. After my birth, my
mother was diagnosed with cancer, and fourteen months later
passed away. I grew up as a child without that mother's physical presence. It has affected me everyday of my life for the past
fifteen years. I grew up as a child confused, I faced the hardships
of elementary school without a mother, and still now every day
I face unanswered questions.

Growing up as a child, I was confused I never really understood
what happened. When I was two my father hired a nanny. She
was there to live and help take care of us. I never thought of her
as a mother, which she wasn't. But just as someone who was
there to look after me. When I was six my nanny, Anna met

someone, got married and moved out. It was hard on my dad a full time job, a six and a nine year old.

One of the biggest things that sticks out in my mind was elementary. I never had that Mom to come and be with me on my first day of school. I can remember every year come Mother's Day the teacher would always make us make gifts. I would always tell them I didn't have a Mom and it shocked them but I said I would make one anyways. Every year as long as I can remember I would take that gift go to my mom's grave and leave it there for her.

I know that it has affected me the most now though. There are so many things I want to know. Now that I am older, I try to understand but it's hard. I just wish I knew what her voice sounded like; I wish I could remember her warm soft touch. I think as I go through adolescence it's the hardest, losing someone too close, too important is the hardest thing as a child. I know as I grow older some of my questions will be answered but there will always be that burning question in my mind. Why?

Thus, growing up through childhood without a mother is hard but it isn't impossible. You need to accept what has happened and move on from there. I myself have learned you can't live your life in the past look at what you have. Things happen for a reason in life. I know I'll meet my mom again one day, but until then I know she loves me and will always be there looking down on me from Heaven's gates.

Jared Lawrence

Part Two
CHIEF

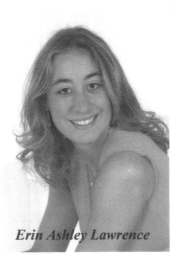

Erin Ashley Lawrence

"The present contains nothing more than the past."
—Henri Bergson

Chapter Five

OUR CHIEF

"We live, we love, we give, but we never give up,
if we give up, we have not accomplished our one goal in life."
—Unknown

Erin had a rare kindness and honesty about her, the kind that made her friends with just about any person she would meet. Like her mother, Erin often wore her personality on her sleeve, and when she smiled her face became the window to her soul. Ever since her mother passed away, she wanted to be a good example for others, so that her mother would be proud of her. In 2000, Erin was fourteen years old and in Grade 8 at St. Josaphat, a Catholic elementary school in northwest Regina. That year Erin received the "Co-operative Spirit of the Prairies," which is awarded annually to the student who:

- Demonstrates a spirit of cooperation, lending a helping hand, and pitching in whenever and wherever help is needed

- Maintains a positive attitude, especially in difficult situations

- Perseveres, even when it would be easier to quit

- Has overcome some adversity, or continues on in the face of adversity, and

- Exemplifies the spirit of the prairie settlers in pulling together regardless of the circumstances.

That was Erin, all right, always putting other people first. It was never about her, but what she could do for you. All that, and tough to boot. Erin had already won an award for perseverance in the face of adversity *before* we found out about the disease.

Sometimes Erin was almost *too* self-effacing. When Erin was younger I always signed her up for sports. She tried all sorts of different sports, but one of her favourites was gymnastics. When Erin was eleven she was interviewed by the Family Channel, which was doing an exposé on youth gymnastics in Canada. The interviewer asked Erin why she had declined to become a competitive gymnast, and her answer was that she *"didn't want to be better than the next person."* Erin never complained much about anything, although sometimes I wish that she had. It wasn't in her to worry about herself; she was too concerned about everyone else. I often wished that, at least sometimes, Erin would put herself first.

Even the best of us are selfish sometimes, but the extraordinary thing about Erin was that selflessness seemed to be her default mode, her natural disposition. Where it is often easiest to put our own needs above those of others, Erin found it difficult to assert herself, even when and where she would be entirely justified in doing so.

Just one example: one day, when Erin was a little girl, she told me that she had a lot of "pimples" on her back and chest, and that they were very itchy. Apparently, this had gone on for three days, without Erin saying anything. Of course, I knew right away that she had the chicken pox.

In 2002, Erin began experiencing stomach problems. I took her to see our family doctor, who prescribed some stomach pills and antacid medication. He had no reason to suspect that it was anything more. Given Erin's age, his diagnosis would probably be shared by most doctors. All the same, I was quite worried at first, but after a couple of weeks of taking the prescribed pills, Erin's stomach seemed to get better. We often hear the cliché that children think they're invincible. From our more worldly perspective as parents, we want to protect them by reminding them that they aren't. But it often goes unspoken that, as parents, many of us often think the very same way; that is to say, because our children are children, we tend to believe that they must be too young to have anything seriously wrong with them. We think we know better, but we can't help thinking that children *ought* to be invincible, that they should be spared the harsh realities that come with adulthood for as long as possible.

My experience with RoseMarie had shattered this illusion, but I couldn't help clinging to it. At the same time, when Erin began to have stomach problems it was impossible for me not to have an unsettling feeling that the past was encroaching upon the present. In 1991, I was told that RoseMarie's cancer was only something that could affect her, and that our children had nothing to worry about. *"You could drink a glass of RoseMarie's cancer and not come down with cancer,"* they said. This wasn't entirely untrue, but as I was to discover, it was also very misleading.

A year passed. Erin was entering her final year of high school when the stomach problems returned. We went back to our family doctor, who prescribed a different type of stomach pill. I knew he was trying to help, but the phrase "same shit different pile" kept coming to mind. I decided I would let the family doctor know of my concerns and make sure that he was aware that Erin's mother had passed away from stomach cancer. It took a bit of convincing, but I managed to get our doctor to write a referral that would send us to a "General and Colorectal" Surgeon by the name of Dr. Malik. Dr. Malik scheduled a gastroscopy for May 7th in the GI Unit at the Pasqua Hospital in Regina, a place I knew ominously well. Both Erin and I were very nervous, but for different reasons: Erin was anxious because she had never been in the hospital before, but I was getting déjà vu.

On the day of Erin's gastroscopy we made our way up to the GI Unit, which was (and still is at the time of writing) housed on the third floor of the Pasqua Hospital. After checking with the desk clerk, a nurse showed us to a private room. There we met with the unit supervisor and head nurse, Lorie McGeough, who also happened to be the mother of one of Erin's friends. Lorie had been a nurse for over twenty years, so I knew Erin would be in good hands. Lorie personally started Erin's IV drip and made us feel as comfortable as possible as we waited for Dr. Malik to arrive.

Dr. Malik, was pleasant and compassionate when I spoke to him about the loss of RoseMarie. Unexpectedly, Dr. Malik asked whether I would be comfortable going in and watching Erin's procedure. I was very surprised, but thought it would be great if I could be there and hold Erin's hand. A few minutes later some nurses arrived with a stretcher and rolled Erin into the procedures room. I noticed the blinds were drawn and the room was mostly dark. Two nurses stood wearing aqua-green hospital scrubs, billowy waterproof isolation gowns, yellow paper facemasks, and what looked like welder's goggles. What slight illumination there was in the room emanated from a bank of glowing monitors attached to a small camera at the end of the scope, which would shortly be winding its way through Erin's esophagus on its way into her stomach. A small plastic clip was placed around the index finger of Erin's right hand to monitor her heart rate, blood pressure, and oxygen levels during the course of the procedure.

Dr. Malik asked Erin to lie on her left side, facing him. He then injected saline solution and Demerol into her IV to relax her. In a few moments Erin's eyes rolled to the top of her head and she was out of it. I remember watching the monitor as Dr. Malik coated the scope with a translucent Xylocaine jelly and gently slid the long black hose down Erin's esophagus. It was the most amazing thing I had ever seen: I was actually looking at the inside of a stomach. It was something like looking at a balloon from the inside. The yellowish tinge of stomach acid and apple-green bile were particularly striking.

Dr. Malik took a series of biopsies (tissue samples): one at the top, one in the middle, and one at the bottom of Erin's stomach. He said that everything seemed to be normal, but that Erin had a considerable amount of bile reflux. We were told that the results would be back in about a week and that Dr. Malik would give us a call. It was the longest week of my life. I was so damned nervous that my own stomach was beginning to bother me. Ten days later, Dr. Malik called and said that everything had came back normal and that he would give Erin a new prescription to help treat her bile reflux.

Things briefly went back to normal. Erin had graduated from high school, and her compassion for other people led her to pursue a future career in psychology. In 2004, Erin began her first year at the University of Regina, entering the Faculty of Arts with a major in psychology. Erin was very studious and took a great deal of responsibility in her career as a student. She was always extra-prepared for exams and papers. If she didn't put one hundred and ten per cent effort into everything, she was never satisfied.

Just prior to entering her third year of University, Erin began to have stomach problems again, which persisted into September. Yet another visit to the family doctor yielded another referral to Dr. Malik, and on December 7th we were back in the GI Unit for another gastroscopy. This time I wasn't asked to come in. I had a dreadful feeling the past was no longer something that could be left behind, but a spectre haunting the present. This time Lorie herself was going into the Procedure Room with Erin. I couldn't hold back my emotions. I hugged Lorie. She had a heart of gold. I told her that if the results for Erin's test turned out bad, *"'Mum's the word."* I could see by the expression on her face that she knew what I meant: I wanted to tell Erin myself.

Dr. Malik took three more biopsies. He thought everything looked normal again, but we would have to wait for the results. Exactly one week later, on December 14th, Dr. Malik's office called and told us that he wanted to see Erin as soon as possible. One of the samples looked "abnormal" and the pathologist was requesting additional biopsies because of the family history.

As with RoseMarie, things began happening very quickly. Dr. Malik insisted that Erin have another scope the following morning. But it was mid-December, which meant that Erin was also in the process of studying for her final exams at the university. Talk about pressure. Yet, Erin never complained. Her finals seemed to be more important to her than her health. The scope would have to wait.

On December 15th, Erin was back for her third scope. I was praying this was nothing more than a contaminated sample or some sort of minor stomach infection. This time, Dr. Malik took over thirty biopsies. He informed us that he wanted the test results shipped to a different lab. Normally it could take up to two weeks to get the results, but because of the Christmas holidays, things would take even longer. It had become clear to me what was going on: he was looking for cancer.

As the sick feeling of this realization shot through me, I prayed I was wrong. Images and voices from sixteen years prior vividly materialized before me. I remembered being told in an assured voice that *"you couldn't get RoseMarie's cancer even if you drank a glass of it."* This probably was a true statement in 1991 because nothing was known about genetic testing or Hereditary Diffuse Gastric Cancer. The thin line that separated the past from the present fluctuated and then dissolved. A cataract of half-forgotten emotions and images started colliding with one another, indiscriminately mixing, throwing time off its axis, out of joint, as if the record of my life had begun to skip, the needle landing again and again on the same spot. The past was in the past, wasn't it? Yet here I was, caught in the vicious circle of a history repeating itself, two different times connected by a single cancerous thread, collapsing into a single moment. This could not happen again. I wouldn't let it happen again.

Chapter Six

FRIENDS AND SOULMATES

"Don't walk behind me; I may not lead. Don't walk in front of me;
I may not follow. Just walk beside me and be my friend."
—Albert Camus

Erin always had a great circle of friends. Her friends and family were probably the most important part of her life. My daughter always had what one might call a "network". She always made time for her friends and would often serve as the mediator between the various little arguments or disputes that would surface every now and then. Erin had a gift for understanding people and being able to help them with their problems. God knows, Erin often had good advice for me whenever I asked for her opinion. She had a very simple approach to the most complex situations: *love*. Erin really did love people and it seemed as though everyone who knew her, loved her back. Although Erin generally defined herself through her selflessness, she had six girlfriends who considered *her* to be very special: Alexandra, Lindsay, Megan, Nicole, Trish, and Lisa.

They always seemed to be together even when they found themselves apart. Each of them had a pet name; it was just their way of being goofy and special to one another. Everyone called Alexandra "Ali". Erin and Ali graduated from high school, played rugby, and went to university together. Lindsay's pet name was "Stupa" (a contraction of her last name). Erin and Lindsay had grown up together as neighbours and playmates. They had been friends since the sandbox and had gone through pretty much everything together, including elementary school and high school. Megan, who had also been Erin's friend through elementary and high school, as well as a soccer teammate, was often referred to as "Megatron."

People always thought that Erin and Nicole – "Nikki" – were sisters, and they loved one another like sisters. These "sisters from a different mister" graduated from elementary and high school together, played rugby and went to university together with the rest of the gang. Erin always told me that Nikki was "the smart one." Trish and Erin graduated from high school, played rugby, went to university, and generally hung out together.

Lisa was Erin's cousin. They grew up together as little girls, played with their first dolls together, and graduated from elementary and high school together. They were more than just cousins they were also best of friends.

Each of them also had their own pet name for Erin. Sometimes Erin was playfully known as "airhead," Lindsay would also refer to her as "Muffin" or "Pumpkin," and Trish called her "Swany" (as in, like a swan. "Swany" apparently came about during a high school gym class in which the girls were supposed to choreograph a dance/gymnastic routine. According to Trish, Erin started doing some strange dance move that looked like a crazy bird flapping its wings). All the guys called her *Chief*, and Chief was the pet name I gave to Erin the day she was born.

But, I wasn't the only important guy in Erin's life who would call her Chief. Erin's best friend was also the love of her life. On March 16, 2002 Erin met a young man named Brett. How they met, and how they came to fall in love, is probably best described in the words of the man himself:

"I first met Erin playing soccer. I don't think we ever spoke ... it was some months later when we first really met at a birthday party. Prior to that night I had spoken with her a few times and I knew that she liked me because her friends wouldn't go a single day without telling me that I should go out with her. I had finally made my mind up while I was snowboarding in Fernie that I was going to ask her out at the birthday party. And the irony was that Erin had just got back from a cruise and she was tired of 'chasing' me if I wasn't interested. So when the girls told her that I liked her she was mad and didn't even want me to ask her anymore. I didn't learn this until long after though. So we were leaving this party early because the birthday girl's parents came home and shut it down, I decided that we should go to my house. Megan drove us there, and on the way I was in the trunk right behind Erin's seat and I remember very clearly being terribly nervous. All of a sudden Megan slammed on the brakes and Erin and I smacked heads. I remember thinking, "there goes your chance, you idiot", but she was cool about it. So once we got to my house we talked all night and realized that we have both been avoiding each other for the previous weeks because we were both pretty shy, and we just talked for hours. The next day I was even more nervous because I planned to ask her out but I didn't know how to do it. So some time in the evening, after a lot of psyching myself up, I got her number

from Megan and phoned her. It was a very short and embarrassing conversation but in the end she said yes and I was so pumped."

Chapter Seven
ANOTHER OPINION

"A friend is equal to love, as love is equal to a friend,
and they both must equal eternity, because eternity never ends."
—Ace Robinson

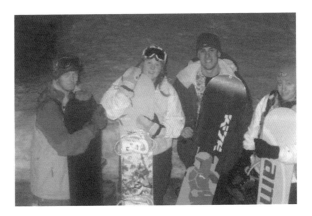

Brett, Lindsay, Tyler, Erin

In the first week of 2007, Erin and some of her friends – Brett, Tyler, Quinn, Lindsay, and Megan – planned a ski trip to Fernie, a small resort city in southeastern British Columbia. Erin borrowed Jared's snowboard and all six of them squeezed into Tyler's midsize SUV and made the nine-hour drive to the Rocky Mountains. Megan decided she wasn't going snowboarding and Quinn only went one day, but Erin, Brett, Tyler and Lindsay would be snowboarding for a full three days. While Erin was away, Dr. Malik's office called and asked that we arrange a time to discuss the results of Erin's biopsies. I knew it couldn't be good news: they wouldn't tell me a thing over the phone. Jan and I arranged to see Dr. Malik that very afternoon.

We sat in a small office for what seemed to like hours. The longer we sat, the closer the walls pressed in. I wanted hope but the walls disapproved. Finally, Dr. Malik appeared in the doorway, looking grave, and everything caved in. "Erin has cancer. Stomach cancer, we think Stage 0 or Stage 1."

Dr. Malik wanted to know when Erin would be returning from Fernie; they needed to operate as soon as possible. We told him that Erin wouldn't be back until late Sunday night. The bitter irony of it crushed me: I would have to tell my daughter, while she was having the time of her life snowboarding down the Rockies, that she had cancer. I couldn't believe it was happening again. I prepared myself, but I didn't yet know what, or how, to tell her. Not a lie, no, but I didn't want to scare her either. The dilemma was familiar to me but no less difficult: how do you tell a loved one they are dying?

When we returned home, we found that Erin had sent us an email.

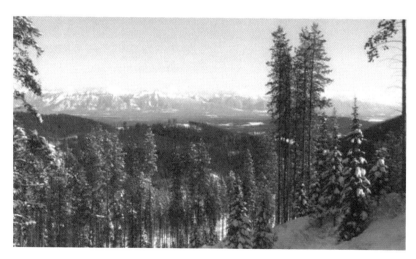

Rockie Mountains

Erin's Gift

January 4, 2007 Fernie, B.C.

Hello Dad,

"O my gosh!!! i love snowboarding! I'm a natural, ahha ok maybe not but im pretty good even Brett and Tyler r impressed with how well and how quickly i learned. I love snowboarding and im definitely doing it again, the mountains are amazing, its beautiful, gods country.

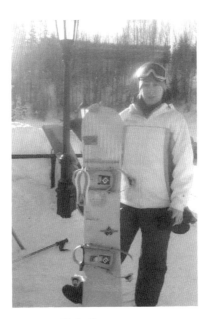

Erin Lawrence

Linds and i sit on the mountain and take a break from boarding cuz the runs are sooo long and we stare at the sun hitting the mountain tops, I'm in love with BC. I thought u might want to know Linds number in case u wanna call. I am having the best time here with everyone we are having so much fun. I am feeling alright, not perfect but pretty good, i take Advil to get rid of the pain in my side and its workin', haha whatever works i gotta keep snowboarding, but overall i've been ok, I hope u got a hold of Dr. Malik so that u can rest at ease. Love you always. and pls dont worry so much about me, mom has my back. love ya tons, Erin Aka Chief"

Just being with friends, having fun, and putting her distressed dad at ease meant more to Erin than her own pain. I was just lying down around 10:00 p.m. on January 7th, when Erin came through the door. I heard some clamour in the garage putting Jared's snowboard away. When she walked into the house she was beaming. "I had the time of my LIFE! Snowboarding is so much fun and the mountains are so beautiful!"

I tried my best to smile. I knew I had to savour this happiness. Erin asked if we had spoken with Dr. Malik and I said that we had. Without waiting to hear the rest of what I had to say, Erin turned and descended the stairs that led to her bedroom and began unpacking her wet ski-pants and jacket.

"So, what did he say?"

I was suddenly unsure of how to continue. Erin turned and looked deeply into my suddenly dumbstruck face, seeing the words I was too afraid to speak.

"It's cancer... I knew it. I just knew it."

I told her what Dr. Malik had told us: the disease was in a very early stage of its development and that, unlike RoseMarie's peritoneal metastasis, Erin's cancer appeared to be relatively contained. There was a chance of removing it through surgery, as long as it was operated upon right away. The next day we went to see our family doctor again, this time to tell him that it was cancer. He shook his head in shock and disbelief and things got very emotional. We informed him that Dr. Malik believed the cancer was at Stage 0 or Stage 1 and that he wanted to operate immediately. We knew time was precious and that we had little to waste, but we let our doctor know we wanted another opinion, ASAP.

I asked for a consultation that would make clear the absolute urgency of the situation. We already had a tentative surgery date and wanted another professional consultation and diagnosis before Erin signed any consent forms and went under the knife. Several patients had mentioned Dr. Carter, an excellent surgeon who would serve as an ideal candidate for a second opinion. I called Dr. Carter's office and told his receptionist over the phone that our situation was desperate. The referral was faxed that day and we waited for Dr. Carter's office to get back to us with an appointment.

A little less than twenty-four hours later, Erin, Jan and myself arrived at Dr. Carter's office. After briefly filling out a questionnaire, the nurses measured Erin's weight, then led the three of us to an examining room. One of Dr. Carter's medical students came in and asked a few questions about Erin's health, previous diagnoses, and symptoms. Shortly afterwards, Dr. Carter entered the office carrying a clipboard. As we explained our situation, Dr.

Carter sat at the opposite end of the room, sometimes interjecting with brief questions, and scribbling notes over the referral from our family doctor.

Dr. Carter then noticed the family history on the questionnaire. After noting Erin's age, Dr. Carter asked what seemed to be a very odd question: "Does Erin have night sweats?" Equally strange, at least to Jan and I, was Erin's response: apparently Erin had been having night sweats for some time.

Some nights, Erin said, she would wake up literally soaked. Jan and I were asked to step out of the room as Dr. Carter examined Erin more closely. When we were invited back in, Dr. Carter said that he agreed with Dr. Malik's assessment: in all likelihood, Erin would need a total gastrectomy. Hoping for some reassurance, we asked Dr. Carter whether this type of surgery was at all common. But Dr. Carter's answer didn't provide anything like reassurance. He informed us that total gastrectomies are not common and that most general surgeons in the city don't do a lot of them. Dr. Carter himself had only performed one surgery of the kind in the last year.

That Friday, we met again with Dr. Malik and Erin signed her consent for a surgery that would involve the total removal of her stomach. Dr. Malik went over the procedure and what we might expect. He mentioned that Erin would be attached to at least one, possibly two, drainage tubes, one that would run out of the side of her abdomen, and potentially one other that would be placed down her esophagus. Both MRI and CAT scan results showed that the cancer had not yet spread beyond the stomach, so Dr. Malik was confident that Erin could be cured through surgery, and that surgery was our only option. Erin put pen to paper and signed the forms.

The past flooded back in and Erin was no longer Erin. Her features gradually transformed into those of her mother. I saw my wife, hunched over a piece of paper, signing her name. I felt the future collapsing. Later, one of the nurses who would be responsible for Erin's care would tell me that if we lived in the past there would be no future. I wondered if there would be a future at all.

Chapter Eight

SURGERY

Erin's surgery was scheduled for Tuesday, January 16th. In the meantime, we tried to go about business as usual. Erin continued to go out with her friends and frequently came home late from Brett's. Since the diagnosis, Erin began having more problems with indigestion and often described having pain on her left side. She could no longer eat without getting sick. A general feeling of discomfort took over. At the time, it felt as though the intervening weekend before the surgery went by like a clock counting backwards. It was Sunday and Erin once again arrived home late from Brett's. I was still awake and went downstairs to talk. She told me that sometimes at night she gets scared and can't sleep.

"But then, I close my eyes and I can sense that Mom's right beside me! I don't feel scared anymore and I can fall asleep. It's happened twice!"

I hadn't been sleeping much either. I let her know about the night before her mother went into surgery that she and I had prayed together for the first time. I thought that if Erin felt her mother near, it might have been something of that prayer echoing through the past to comfort us in the present.

The night before Erin was to have her surgery, she came home late again from Brett's. I heard her come through the front door and scramble downstairs. I waited a few minutes for Erin to change and then went down. I knocked at the door and heard a muffled voice tell me to 'come in.' Erin was standing with her back towards me, facing her closet hanging up her clothes. When she turned I could see that she had been crying. I gave her a big hug and told her that I loved her. We could both feel the fear within each of ourselves, surging like an electric current. We were both scared to death. That night I did something I hadn't done since Erin was just a little girl: I lay beside her and held her.

51

Neither of us could sleep and tomorrow was only a few hours away. It was a night I will remember the rest of my life. We shared tears of the past and tears of the present. I couldn't tell Erin my fears. She was too young to remember her mother being sick and I didn't want to make any comparisons for her. We tried to stay positive. Dr. Malik said that surgery was a potential cure. I remember looking at the clock on Erin's dresser and counting down the hours. We had to get ready to go to the hospital at 7:00 a.m., Erin's surgery was scheduled for 8:00 a.m.

I got up just before 7:00 a.m. packed the car and put together a bag for Erin to use while she was in the hospital. We said goodbye to Jared and left around 7:15 a.m. Jan drove, while I sat in the back seat with Erin. Erin said that the pains in her stomach were getting worse. I held Erin's hand while she kept repeating over and over, "I just want to get rid of it! I just want it to go away!"

We arrived at the hospital shortly before 7:30 a.m. and already the waiting room was full of people, so we took a number and waited to be called. The clock had reached a quarter to eight when the O.R called down to Admitting and said that they were waiting for Erin Lawrence in Surgery, and we were processed immediately. They slapped a plastic wristband on her, shoved some files together, and sent us upstairs. A nurse met us in the Preadmission Clinic for the OR and, after checking Erin's wristband, led us to a separate room where they had her change into a hospital gown. Erin stuffed her clothes into a large plastic bag and handed me her glasses. Like RoseMarie, Erin was blind without them. Shadows everywhere. Shadows everywhere, again. A nurse started an IV and gave Erin a pill to help her relax. I think I needed one as well. The nurses told us that Erin wouldn't be out of surgery until around 1:00 p.m. so it would be better if Jan and I went home.

I was beginning to get déjà vu again. I was having problems separating the past from the present into neat compartments. Everything was a reminder. I didn't think it possible that things like this could happen twice in a lifetime. Everything, *everything*, seemed to be a mere repetition of what had happened with RoseMarie, like I was caught in a Ecclesiastical nightmare: "there is nothing new under the sun." The cruelty of it was that I was completely lucid, completely aware. I wasn't losing it, I wasn't going mad, I wasn't trapped inside of a dream. I kept coming back to the cold truth that this was happening, that this was all too real. We drove home, but my mind was still behind me, at the hospital.

I couldn't help thinking about how Erin too, was blind without her glasses. Shadows obscuring things even in the blaring light of the noonday sun, which, to my fevered mind, began to dissolve into the amplified blaze of wall-mounted surgery lamps.

When we arrived back home Jared had already left for school. He was entering his final semester of Grade 12 at Riffel, the same school his sister had graduated from two years before. Although it was still bright outside I lit a candle and placed it on the kitchen table. I was truly afraid. I wanted it to represent the Holy Spirit, I wanted it to burn away the past, to exterminate its long shadow over the present.

I sat in the living room crying and shaking and praying as the clock chimed out the hours. At some point during the day, I don't remember when, I wandered down to Erin's room and down on her bed. The sheets were still wrinkled with the outline of where I had held her the night before. I noticed something sitting on the corner table that I had not seen when I was downstairs earlier to fetch Erin's bag. It was an envelope. "DAD" was written in blue ink across the front. I thought Erin must have placed it there right before we left for the hospital. I reached over, nervous and shaking inside, and opened it. As I read the words, I could hear Erin's voice.

Jan.11/07

Dear Dad,

"I know how worrisome and stressful this time has been for you and will continue to be until I am healthy again. Actually, I probably have no idea of the real agony you are experiencing but if it puts your mind to ease at all, I'm not worried! I have the best support system anyone could ever hope for. I had no idea what an impact my life has had thus far on you and I'm overwhelmed by it all. You always say I only deserve the best at everything in life and that nothing less than the best is good enough! But you failed to realize I already have the best! There is no greater father in the world than you! In no way am I exaggerating, you are the most remarkable and selfless person I have ever met in my 20 yrs. I truly am the luckiest girl in the world to have been blessed with you as my father. And as you're reading this please don't disregard what you've just read, it is the truth. You truly have saved my life because if it were not for you I still would not have been diagnosed. You've told me it was God who saved me and you're right; but you've failed to realize God has worked through you to save my life. The hardest part is over. I'm having surgery probably as you're reading this and when it's over I'll come out better than before. Words

do not exist to describe how thankful I am to you for everything and just how much I love you! Life will go on and someday I'm going to make you a Grandpa so please remember to take care of yourself too! See you when I'm out of surgery and remember God's working through you! And I promise I'll be around forever.

Love you always,"

'Chief'

I had barely finished reading Erin's letter when the phone rang, screaming through the silence like a nuclear siren. It was only 12:15 p.m. and the hospital was already calling to say that Dr. Malik wanted to meet with us. I had this terrifying feeling. I could only hope that he had finished ahead of schedule and just wanted to discuss the surgery. I felt I always had to keep positive. Despair was everywhere, entropy creeping within every nook, reminding me. I resolved to steal myself against despair, against death. Whatever came next, Erin and I would meet it head on.

This time it was my turn to drive and I couldn't get there fast enough. I drove as if the devil himself was on my tail. Despite wanting to keep my emotions in check, I was in a fury. I was shaking by the time we arrived at the hospital. The nurses were talking and whispering with one another as Jan and I raced into the OR. I had one of those feelings you get when you notice that everyone knows something that you don't. Something was definitely wrong. Jan and I were escorted to a private room and told that Dr. Malik would be in to speak with us shortly.

I was trembling and praying that my worst fears were not coming true. I was hoping against hope itself that I was only overreacting. When Dr. Malik finally arrived he didn't come alone. He sank heavily into his chair and introduced us to one of the hospital's social workers. I looked Dr. Malik in the eyes, but he began to shake his head in disappointment and disbelief.

"I'm sorry... I'm so sorry, and I just can't believe it. I've never seen such an aggressive form of stomach cancer. She's so young, it's already at Stage 4. We were ready to remove the stomach, had her clamped off and couldn't do it. The cancer had spread to the gullet and she would have bled to death on the table. I called Dr. Gorman in to get another opinion. He agreed with me. We left the stomach in and did what we thought would be best for Erin. She will have to have chemo right away after she recovers from surgery."

Jan collapsed. The social worker lunged to keep her steady. I was in total shock and for a moment I couldn't even see. I could not believe what I had just heard. I couldn't believe that we were just told that Erin is going to die of stomach cancer. This was not what we were told going into surgery. The disease was supposed to be at Stage 0 or Stage 1.

Dr. Malik just kept shaking his head and told us that the CT scan had looked normal and that nothing in the results would have led him to suspect anything like this. I could see he had tears in his eyes, and it seemed as though Dr. Malik was experiencing just as much shock and pain as we were. He told us for the first time that he too had a twenty-year-old daughter. I asked that the hospital supply me with a cot. I wasn't leaving Erin's bedside until she was fit enough to come home. Dr. Malik made all the necessary arrangements.

Chapter Nine

RECOVERY

"A physician can sometimes parry the scythe of death,
but has no power over the sand in the hourglass."
—Hester Piozzi Thrale

Before we left the hospital we were told that Erin wouldn't be back from the Recovery Room until 4:00 p.m. Jan asked if I was okay to drive and I said that I was. Jared had been writing his final exams that week and was already home when we got back. I was still taking off my boots when Jared came to the front door and asked me how the surgery went. He could see that we had been crying our eyes out. I told him that they couldn't remove Erin's stomach because the cancer had spread too quickly, that the disease had already reached Stage 4, and that Erin would have to have chemo as soon as she recovered from surgery.

Jared is a very strong young man and often keeps his emotions to himself, but not today. I can count the number of times I've seen Jared cry on one hand since his mother passed away, and I had only ever seen him weep openly when we would visit RoseMarie's grave. This time it was different, this time we felt and shared in one another's pain. He lost his mother before he was old enough to remember her. Now his sister was dying. I told him that Erin's prognosis wasn't good, but that we were a family and families stick together. We would be there to support Erin, no matter what.

Jared decided he couldn't visit Erin right away and I understood. He had to come to grips with what was happening on his own terms, and said he would come up later in the evening. Jan and I went back to the hospital around 3:15 p.m. but Erin still was not down from recovery. I felt some relief that we had arrived before Dr. Malik had the chance to speak to Erin about her surgery; I wanted to be the one to tell her.

Flashbacks crept up on me again. I saw myself standing again in dim light, telling RoseMarie that they didn't get all the cancer. This time I had to tell her daughter the same thing. The only difference was that Erin wouldn't be having two-thirds of her stomach removed. Otherwise, Erin was in the same hospital, on the same ward, and had just undergone the same surgery as her mother sixteen years before, even after the doctors said it could never happen.

I felt I was passing in and out of hallucination. I felt I couldn't hold on to my mind much longer. I wanted to pinch myself just to see if I could snap out of the nightmare. I wished that things had been different, that my life was different. But these were just wishes. The reality of it is this and nothing more than this. I was forty-six years old. My wife passed away sixteen years ago from stomach cancer, and today my twenty-year-old daughter has Stage 4 cancer of the stomach. The facts were like jagged bits of glass, digging into my brain, pieces of a shattered family photo that we never had the chance to take.

It was around 4:30 in the afternoon when they brought Erin down from recovery on a stretcher. She was barely conscious and could hardly open her eyes. Her mouth was so dry small flecks of dried spittle clung to the corners of her mouth, and her voice had shriveled almost to nothing, a hoarse whisper. I grabbed hold of her hand to let her know I was there. It would still be a few more hours before Erin would regain consciousness.

I was hoping when Erin woke up she wasn't going to ask the same question her mother had asked me. I wasn't ready to discuss Erin's prognosis yet. I prayed to God, *I need more time. She needs more time.* I thought that God had helped me that night. He would grant more time. Erin had never been under anesthetic before and was pretty groggy – in no state to hear what I needed to tell her. Erin spent the rest of the night going in and out of sleep. I don't think she remembered when Jared came to visit, and she didn't seem to know what day it was. When she did briefly speak, she asked what time it was and if it was Wednesday, and I told her it was still Tuesday night.

After a while, I sent Jan and Jared home and told them I would stay in the hospital with Erin. I lay on a hard cot beside Erin's hospital bed, but I wouldn't sleep that night. I kept looking at Erin and seeing her mother. She had her mother's personality and looks, but she now had her cancer, a devastating inheritance. I held her hand as she slept.

I remembered from RoseMarie's surgery that Erin would be in a great deal of pain for the next few days. I knew what to expect, I knew that the doctors seemed to know just as little about the disease as they did sixteen years ago. It couldn't be detected and when it was detected, it was too late. All I knew for certain was that I wasn't going to lie to Erin. But I also promised myself that I wasn't going to take her hope away by telling her what the doctors were telling me; namely, that Erin had very little time left and had very little chance at survival. I was caught between mutually exclusive promises, neither of which I could break. I couldn't lie and I couldn't bring myself to tell the truth. What I wouldn't do I had already done. What I had to do I couldn't. No exit.

The next day Erin was more coherent and began to talk. I asked her how much pain she was having on a scale of 1–10, one being the least and ten being the most. Erin said that she wasn't completely sure. Erin didn't really know how to define the pain, since she had never had any kind of surgery before. She was certainly having some pain, so it was definitely not a one, but she wasn't pulling out her hair in agony either, so it wasn't a 10. Erin decided that the pain was perhaps around 3 or 4, and I was glad to hear it. I decided then that I would tell her what we knew and what had happened.

I held her hand and told her that the cancer wasn't at Stage 0 or 1, that when Dr. Malik opened her up, he found that the cancer was more aggressive than had been anticipated, and that it had spread all the way through the lining of her stomach. The disease was up to Stage 4, and she would need chemo when she recovered from surgery. I thought that was enough information for Erin at that particular moment. I didn't want to tell Erin everything, especially that Dr. Malik had left her stomach in place. I still had to figure out how to lay that bombshell.

I knew that I had to find some way to tell her before Dr. Malik came to see her. He said he would be around on Thursday or Friday, so the next morning, after the nurses made their rounds, I made a point of talking with Erin about her prognosis. When I asked Erin how she was feeling the next day, she said her chest was very sore, and she was having trouble taking deep breaths. I explained that her chest was so sore because the surgeons had to cut through her chest muscles in order to access the stomach. After a pause, I told Erin that Dr. Malik had decided not to remove her stomach. There was a vacuum of silence. I will never forget the look on Erin's face. She stared straight into me and in a stern voice said, *"You're kidding me, right?"*

I said that I was serious. I explained that the doctors couldn't remove her stomach because the cancer had spread too high into the gullet. Any attempt at removing it and Erin would have likely died right there on the table. Our only option was to begin chemo and destroy enough cancer cells so that the next time they could successfully remove her stomach. Almost in tears, Erin said, "You mean I have to go through all this again?"

I recalled what Dr. Malik had said to me: surgically, there was nothing he could do to get rid of Erin's cancer. I then remembered something that Erin once said to me when she was younger about people who were terminally ill: "You should never tell anyone that they're dying, or tell someone that they only have so long to live. It's not their decision. It's God's decision."

I decided to answer Erin's question using her own philosophy. I told her that someday she would have another surgery, but first things first: we had to let the chemo destroy her cancer. Erin wasn't very impressed. "You mean I went through all of this for nothing?"

But the surgery wasn't completely for nothing. Dr. Malik had surgically implanted what's known as a "J-Tube" and a "Port-A-Cath." The J-Tube would supplement Erin's nutrition through an external food pump, while the Port-A-Cath, a small medical appliance installed beneath the skin in the upper chest just beneath the collarbone, would allow drugs to be injected and multiple blood samples taken without the discomfort of repeated "needle sticks."

The next day Erin had special visitors. Jared and Jan were visiting every day, but today Brett had come up with his parents Lyn and Grant. It was great to see them. Brett was a special kind of guy. I noticed that while Brett was there Erin lit up like a 100-watt bulb. I could tell they were very much in love. After visiting hours were over, I escorted Brett, Lyn and Grant to the elevator. Before they left I took Brett aside. I had to make sure he was fully aware of Erin's condition. He said that he wasn't going to leave her and that he was going to help Erin fight the disease until the very end. He said he loved her and that wasn't going to change because she had cancer. I have to say my admiration for this young man increased a hundredfold over the course of Erin's illness. His strength and resolve reminded me of the strength I had found in myself when RoseMarie passed away, and I knew we were going to be a team.

I began to cry when I told him about Erin's mother, that she had passed away of the same disease in 1991.

Three days later, Erin had to get up and stand for the first time since the surgery. Two nurses came into the room, checked Erin's dressings and prepared a sponge bath, while I went for a walk. I tried once more to regain composure. I walked the halls trying to sort things out. I knew the nurses planned to get Erin up and walking after her sponge bath and remembered the pain that RoseMarie had to endure in her first time walking after surgery. I felt scared for Erin. I kept telling myself I had to keep positive and supportive for Erin. I had to keep down the irrational but persistent feeling that my family was under some kind of curse.

As I wandered the halls my mind wandered between exhortations of prayer and complete despondency: *Never say never and the answer is no unless you ask, right Lord? Ok, I'm asking I'm asking for a miracle, not for me, but for Erin. RoseMarie told me she would always be there for the children. I can't think of a better time than now. First RoseMarie, and now Erin. It's too much to believe, it's too much to handle, Lord it's a living nightmare, and I can't do a damn thing about it!*

As I wandered, I thought I recognized a colleague of Dr. Malik's who had assisted with Erin's surgery. I introduced myself as Erin's dad and right away he lowered his eyes, saying that he was sorry, so sorry, Erin was so young. I asked him how long he thought my daughter had to live and I noticed tears began welling in his eyes.

"Not long, not very long."

"How long?"

"Maybe six months." He said that he already knew, and that he was sorry. I remembered when we were told that RoseMarie had only six months to live. They were wrong: she lived seven. That probably doesn't seem like much to get excited about, but when you're told you only have a few months to live and you're living day to day, another month is a very big deal. I said that I hoped he was wrong. He cupped his hand on my shoulder and said, "Me too."

Erin was looking perky and sitting up in her bed when I got back to the room. She was practicing pulling herself up with a T-Bar that was now attached to a metal frame around the hospital bed. After a few minutes, she said it felt as though there was no strength left in her muscles. The muscles in her abdomen and chest had been cut apart, and it would take a quite a long time for these things to heal. I let Erin know that the nurses were already on their way back to help her get out of bed. In a familiar tone, Erin stared me down and said, "You've *got* to be joking."

I said I wasn't and the first time would hurt like a son-of-a-bitch, but that the more often she got up, the easier it would eventually become.

"You think so?" she asked.

I told her that I didn't think, I knew.

"You know Dad, I don't know what I would do without you! You stay in the hospital with me all the time. You sleep in a cot beside me. I'm never alone, I'm not scared... I'm glad you're here."

"I wouldn't want to be anywhere else."

"I owe you big time, pops."

"You don't owe me a thing, Chief."

Erin asked how Jared was doing at school and I told her that he had an exam that morning and another one in the afternoon, but after that he would be coming up with Jan. Then the nurses came back in to get Erin out of bed for her first walk. They asked where Erin's pain was at, and she told them it was about a '4'. The nurses checked the pain medication in her epidural and decided to try standing her up right next to the bed, just as a start. They helped Erin swing her legs over the bed and transferred her catheter to a portable IV pole. Erin lurched forward, grasping at the nurses to support her weakened frame. Erin began to shake violently as her feet touched the floor, and her face suddenly blanched.

"I think I'm gonna pass out..."

The nurses braced themselves and guided Erin back onto the bed, their three bodies jerking around one another in a strange dance. I ran for a wet face cloth and dabbed Erin's forehead until the colour began returning to her face. The nurses said unsteadiness was quite common and probably due to the epidural, which can slow the heart rate and often made a person feel weak. They said we would try a walk again tomorrow. In the meantime, Dr. Malik had ordered Heparin injections once a day to prevent blood clots from forming in Erin's legs.

At night, a nurse would wrap Erin's legs in special cuffs to help with circulation. These cuffs are very similar to the kind of armbands one would use to measure blood pressure, except that they are wrapped around the calf muscles instead of the upper arm. The cuff circulates hot or cool air, inflating and deflating automatically to help stimulate the blood and reduce the risk of clotting. They told us that the epidural couldn't be removed until Erin was up and walking on a regular basis. I joked that, the catheter would be Erin's best friend for now: she should savour not having to get out of bed every time she needed to go to the bathroom. I saw a faint smile cross her lips and both of us prepared for another long night.

Erin really liked Arnie, the night nurse. Arnie always made his rounds using a small flashlight so as not to disturb the patients, he would always be in checking up on Erin's temperature, changing her IV bags, making sure her food pump was working properly, and draining her catheter.

The next day, Erin was determined to get out of bed by herself and wanted her catheter removed. The same two nurses from yesterday were both working the day shift again, and once again they came together to help Erin make a second attempt at walking. Using the T-bar hanging above the bed, Erin pulled herself forward, and with the help of the nurses swung her legs over the side. I put a pair of slippers on Erin's feet while she very slowly, very painfully, put pressure on her legs and stood up. For the second time, Erin's upper body began to shake as her ravaged abdominal muscles tried to sustain the weight of her body. And for the second time Erin turned white as a ghost. She found it very difficult to breathe and wasn't able to take any deep breaths when the nurses asked her to.

Slowly Erin shuffled her legs, leaning onto her IV pole, which rattled and creaked as the wheels inched forward. We escorted Erin out of her room. The nurses were glad to see Erin up and about. One of them made a joke about how nurses often celebrate things that most of us would find a bit strange.

"When you're able to pass gas we clap!"

"When you have a bowel movement we throw a party!"

It was a sign, the nurses said, that the body was beginning to wake up, and that the digestive system was beginning to work again. When the body is bedridden and immobile, one develops a lot of gas, and walking helps to relieve stomach cramps. It might sound a bit vulgar, but after gastric surgery, a "fart" is something grand.

We went for a walk twice that day and each time Erin found it a little easier to get out of bed. The nurses kept a close eye on the amount of fluids Erin consumed during the day, and would measure this amount alongside the quantity of urine in her catheter. This would tell them that Erin's kidneys were still working properly. Only two days after her surgery, Erin was already walking and expelling a good ratio of fluids. Her kidneys appeared to be working fine and Dr. Malik told the nurses they could remove her catheter. This was quite an accomplishment: passing gas, walking around, and getting your catheter out all on the same day, so soon after surgery.

A short time later, Erin and I went for a good long walk. We walked at least twenty minutes, making a double loop around the hospital ward. We had just walked through the TV lounge area when Erin stopped and said that she really felt strange. I saw that her face had gone snow-white again and I looked around hoping to see someone else in the lounge, but it was empty. We needed a chair but I couldn't leave Erin alone long enough to find one. I was supporting Erin by her left arm and I didn't want to leave her standing alone in the hallway. All of a sudden, she collapsed.

I tried to grab hold of her before her head hit the floor. I had one arm hooked under her armpit and tried to brace her against my legs, but she dropped so instantly that there was little I could do. The IV pole crashed on top of us and we both fell to the floor in a heap. I began screaming for help. Thankfully, a nurse at the other end of the hall heard me and rushed over to us. The nurse began yelling *"Code Blue!"* – the code for a cardiac arrest – and four more nurses were at our side almost instantaneously. Erin was still out cold as they checked her pulse and tried to determine whether her pupils were dilated. A minute later, an eternity as far as I was concerned, Erin's eyes began to flutter and she slowly regained consciousness.

Dr. Malik was notified and he told the nurses he wanted Erin's epidural removed the next morning. An Automatic Pain Control (APC) pump was ordered that day and Erin's pain medication was changed to Hydromorphone. I asked what that was and I was told it is six times stronger than Morphine. I asked the nurses to explain why Erin had passed out. They told me that an epidural is ideal for pain control while a person is bedridden, but not very good for the body after a person becomes mobile.

Because the epidural considerably lowers both heart rate and blood pressure, when Erin began walking, the heart couldn't get enough oxygen to the brain, causing Erin to pass out. After they removed the epidural, the nurse explained, there was a considerably lower risk of Erin passing out again. We would still need to take several walks each day, building up her atrophied muscles, until Erin was comfortable getting out of bed without assistance.

Dr. Malik stopped by almost every day to monitor Erin's progress. On one of his visits he informed us that he had referred Erin to the Allan Blair Cancer Centre. He did not want to discharge Erin from the hospital until she had an appointment to see an oncologist who would help us plan continued treatment.

This brings us to about January 19th. While I was staying in the hospital with Erin, Jan was at home with Jared. Most nights she found herself overwhelmed with phone calls, answering the same questions over and over. Jan was up late every night hammering away on the computer answering e-mails and conversing with friends anxious to know what was happening, how things were developing, if Erin was getting better, how we were all hanging in there.

This particular night was different. Jan was searching the Canadian Cancer Society website for something, anything, that could tell us more about Erin's cancer and couldn't come up with anything. Eventually, Jan happened across a link that led to a doctor by the name of David Huntsman, a Genetic Pathologist who worked at the Centre for Translational and Applied Genomics (CTAG) for the B.C. Cancer Agency in Vancouver. Jan discovered that Dr. Huntsman and his colleagues had developed a blood test to screen for the mutated gene said to be at the root of Hereditary Diffuse Gastric Cancer (CDH1).

Jan immediately e-mailed Dr. Huntsman and explained what had happened to RoseMarie and now, to Erin. Much to our surprise, Dr. Huntsman replied the very next morning. He suggested that Erin should have a blood test to determine if she was carrying the CDH1 genetic mutation. If this was the case, Dr. Huntsman averred, then other family members would have the option of being tested as well. Jan immediately drove to the hospital to inform me of our good fortune and to discuss what we could do next. That same day, Dr. Malik brought someone with him on his regular visit to Erin's room.

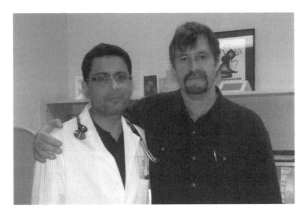

Dr. Aboo and myself

We were introduced to Dr. Aboo, Erin's oncologist at the Allan Blair Cancer Centre. Dr. Aboo came highly recommended. Dr. Malik described him as a young and aggressive doctor who was 'up to snuff' with the latest developments in chemotherapy. Through his spirited approach to research, Dr. Aboo would try to find the most aggressive cancer treatments available at the time.

I knew Dr. Malik wanted the best treatment and care for Erin. I knew he felt terrible about the prognosis and he was doing his best to ensure Erin never fell through any cracks in the system. He wanted Erin prioritized even when she wasn't directly under his care. We all knew that time was not on Erin's side. Yet she needed more time, time to heal physically from her surgery before we could start anything too aggressive in terms of chemotherapy.

Dr. Aboo feared that entering chemo too soon would not only destroy the cancer but disrupt the healing process as well, possibly reopening the incision from her surgery. This would obviously be a giant setback, and potentially fatal. Nevertheless, Dr. Aboo said he hoped they could begin treatments approximately two weeks after Erin was to be discharged.

Erin and I spent the next ten days in the hospital. I will treasure this time forever. As hospital roomies, we spent some real quality time together. We talked about RoseMarie and Erin asked me how she passed away. I told her the truth: after RoseMarie's stomach was removed she could no longer hold anything down, and as a result, she starved to death. Erin asked if that would happen to her. I said that it didn't seem likely. RoseMarie had never been given a J-tube that would consistently stream a food supplement into her, keeping her body going. RoseMarie had never even had the option. I lost her to this disease and, God help us, we weren't going to lose Erin too. Chief promised me she wasn't going anywhere. Not once did Erin ever think she couldn't beat the disease.

I found some comfort in this, but it was just too painful to think about the alternative. I promised myself, as a favour to Erin, that I would never speak in negative terms about anything having to do with the disease. I remembered the letter she had written to me before she went in for surgery: Erin believed I saved her life. But right then I felt I hadn't done anything of the kind. Sixteen years ago, I dropped the ball. I should have learned something about the disease when I lost RoseMarie. Now it seemed only God could help us. I wasn't going to tell Erin what the doctors had told me. I thought Erin was right, it wasn't our place to tell a dying person how long they have to live, it was God's decision... wasn't it?

If it wasn't, then we were living in a world that was nothing but directionless chaos, without anything like meaning or hope. The disease was an agent of this chaos.

What is cancer, really? Uncontrollable growth. Invasion. An *obscenity*. A "noisome pestilence" that both "walketh in darkness" and "wasteth at noonday." What can it mean that such a thing can *be*? If God created cancer, he created it in anger. Cancer exists for no reason other than its own reproduction. It is the dark glass, the inverted reflection, of Erin's selflessness. Cancer strikes me as what life becomes when it exists only in and for itself; a selfish, swarming, destructive form of life. The thought is lonely and terrifying for me, I refuse it. We are all born to die. Some of us are only here for a short period of time. Life's a gift and we should not take it for granted. There is a song that says *only the good die young.* I thought I really believed that. But it still scares me. The disease still scares the shit right out of me.

My Chief is a better person than I will ever be. She never thinks of herself. Her only concern is for others. Erin has so much character, so much life. Everyone who knows her loves her. I love her. I love my daughter and I need her in my life.

When I lost RoseMarie to the disease in 1991, I prayed for a miracle. I now prayed for another. This time things will be, no, they *have to be*, different. I asked God to grant to Erin the miracle that RoseMarie never received. I would have never believed this could happen twice in my family. They say lightning never strikes twice in the same location. But cancer is anarchy, flouting every law of nature. It can wipe out entire families, destroy the ones you love, and change your life forever.

Chapter Ten

CONSULTATION

"Things turn out best for the people who
make the best of the way things turn out."
—Art Linkletter

The last time I visited the Allan Blair Cancer Centre I was with RoseMarie in September of 1990. Since then, the Centre had been completely renovated and redesigned. There was a new reception area, separate private offices for social workers as well as a newly completed and much needed chemo treatment area. This was far superior to the old section of the Pasqua Hospital Ward 2E, which all those years ago had resembled a set from the movie *"Escape from Alcatraz."* Erin, Brett, Jan and I made our way into the clinic. I had decided Jared should not be there for obvious reasons. Erin was still in a wheelchair, recovering from surgery.

We were taken to a private room where a nurse asked what seemed like a pretty stupid question about whether there was any history of cancer in the family. We had been asked this question so many times by so many people that I was always surprised everyone didn't already know. After a short time, the nurse asked us if we had any questions for her, and that was opening Pandora's Box.

We drilled her with questions regarding why we weren't informed about the possibility that the disease was genetic, and why they didn't already know that I had had two children with RoseMarie. The nurse was speechless. I thought she shouldn't be asking questions if she couldn't even answer ours. We made our way back to the waiting area and met with Dr. Aboo's nurse, Mardel, who directed us to a cramped examination room. Dr. Aboo sidled into the room after us, trying to negotiate around the wheelchair, Erin, the nurse, and myself in the rapidly contracting space, carrying a clipboard and Erin's medical records. I noticed that Dr. Aboo was dressed very professionally, wearing a long white overcoat, dress shirt, and tie.

Erin and I had met him once before, but for Jan and Brett this was the first time. I was impressed, and encouraged by Dr. Aboo's demeanour and his professionalism. Coupled with Dr. Malik's description of Dr. Aboo's youthful vigour, his confidence, and his knowledge of the latest research on chemotherapy, we all knew that he would be the right oncologist for Erin.

But at that time, there was very little research available on the disease and as a result, a zero success rate in treatment. Regardless, I was glad we were with someone who would put us on the offensive. Dr. Aboo was very pleasant and made his best attempt to leave us with a positive attitude. He offered Erin an "aggressive" treatment plan in the form of chemotherapy that would combine drug infusion with possible radiation treatment. The drug regimen involved the injection of three separate chemo drugs: Epirubicin, Cisplatin, and Fluorouracil (5FU), or "ECF" for short. The drugs would either be administered through a thin plastic cannula inserted just beneath the skin and into a vein near the collarbone, or through a PICC line inserted into the crook of the arm. The Epirubicin, which bore the deep red of wine or blood, would be first given as an injection or infusion along with a saline drip. The Cisplatin, colourless but slightly opaque, would follow. Once completed, a portable pump, small enough to clip to a belt loop or pocket, would be attached to the line to begin releasing a controlled dose of 5FU into the bloodstream.

The whole process would have to be repeated, the drug reservoirs or the pump itself replaced, on a weekly basis. Dr. Aboo also recommended that Erin be referred to an outside centre that had a surgeon with more expertise in dealing with this kind of situation. He also suggested that an inquiry be made through the Mayo Clinic or some other centres to see if they had anything else to offer in the way of treatment. There was the possibility of using a trial drug called Herceptin, an antibody normally associated with treating breast cancer. Future tests would determine if Erin's HER-2/neu receptor, a protein that regulates cell growth, was defective. I remember asking what this meant.

Dr. Aboo explained that if Erin tested positive for this certain protein that is produced by some types of cancer, they would have to use a different treatment protocol. Dr. Aboo informed us that less than one per cent of the population develops gastric cancer before the age of twenty. One in three patients are treated successfully and their cancer forced into remission.

We discussed my concerns for Jared and Dr. Aboo promised that he would immediately make a consultation visit with Dr. Edmond Lemire, a doctor who specializes in genetics and practices in Saskatoon, a city about two hundred and thirty kilometres northwest of Regina. We spoke of the possibility that some of our extended family members would also have to undergo genetic testing. The three of us were then escorted into a more comfortable lounge area where Mardel discussed Erin's treatment in more detail, letting us know about the risks and possible side effects of each of the drugs she would be taking.

Everybody reacts to chemo in different ways. Some don't experience any side effects, but the drugs can reduce the production of both white and red blood cells, increasing the risk of anemia and infection. Nausea, fatigue, hair loss, dry skin, ringing in the ears, tingling in the hands or feet (neuropathy), dry mouth, sore mouth, ulcers, diarrhea, rounded out the list of casualties of a body at war with itself. We asked as many questions as we could think of. Mardel was extremely compassionate and answered as best she could.

Over the next week, Erin was booked for a CAT scan, an MRI (magnetic resonance imaging) and an echocardiogram (ECG). They never told us why she needed these tests, but I didn't have to be a doctor to figure out what they were doing. I had been through all of this before. I was hoping chemotherapy would be more effective in controlling the disease than what had happened sixteen years earlier with RoseMarie. Because we were dealing with a rare form of hereditary stomach cancer, the doctors had to establish a "baseline."

The ECG would determine if Erin's heart was strong enough for such an aggressive form of chemo. I wondered if they could hook me up to the leads. I didn't know if my heart was strong enough to go through it all again. It would have to be. Dr. Aboo had assured us that this treatment would give Erin her best chance of survival and quality of life. Dr. Aboo scheduled a follow-up consultation for February 6th at 2:00 p.m. to confirm Erin's treatments before chemo was to begin.

On January 26th, we checked out of the hospital. The next thing was to make arrangements and get a hold of a food pump, but I wasn't able to obtain a requisition for the pump from the Saskatchewan Abilities Council. Erin needed a pump right away, but going through the regular channels would take a few weeks. The administrator from the ward was a great guy and totally compassionate. He made arrangements to give us a loaner. I paid a deposit, and we were good to go.

It was a weird feeling walking out of the hospital pushing Erin in a wheelchair. All the nurses came to say goodbye and wished Erin all the best in her treatment. Erin had made so many friends during her stay. We had so many flowers we couldn't take them all home with us, so we gave most of them to the nurses. Jared pulled the family car to the front doors of the hospital. Brett and I packed Erin's food pump and IV pole into the car, loaded the rest of the flowers, gifts, and packages into the trunk, and drove off.

Chapter Eleven
CHEMO

"Life is too short to live the same day twice."
—Anonymous

On February 7th, Erin, Brett, and I went together for Erin's first chemo session. It was a little before our 8:00 a.m. appointment and we all sat nervously in the near empty waiting area. I never enjoyed watching RoseMarie go through her treatments and I wasn't looking forward to watching my daughter go through the same thing. I was tortured by memories of the past. Unbidden, they began to seep through the clean white paint and I felt the old prison atmosphere of Ward 2E welling up around me. Despite the facelift, I could feel the same pallid gloom from sixteen years prior. It hung about the place like a stink.

They called us when Erin's 'chair' was ready. We were escorted down a narrow hallway that led us past the children's chemo area. Erin's jaw dropped. She gripped my arm and said, "Oh my God, Dad... that's terrible!"

Erin's first thought was about how awful it was for those children, and not how she was about to become a part of that same world, that she herself was still just a child. Five minutes away from her first chemo treatment, and it was still all about others' suffering, not her own. We walked into the chemo ward and I was immediately overwhelmed by a large number of recliner chairs situated along the walls. It was shortly after 8:00 a.m. and the area was now almost full of patients. The first thing I noticed was that Erin was the youngest person they had in chemo that day. I kept having the feeling *we should not be here.* The question *why me, why us?* kept repeating itself over and over in my head. I wondered if Erin was having the same thoughts but there were no outward signs. Like her mother, Erin never complained about anything. Regardless, everyone sitting in a recliner that morning had one thing in common. It was not their choice to be here. They were all fighting the disease and hoping to increase their odds of survival.

Despite the substantial number of people in the room, it was extremely quiet. There had to be at least thirty of us. Some were sleeping in their recliners, others were watching television, listening to a Walkman, or reading. I remember they gave Erin chair #5 because it was part of my birth date. Erin sat down as we were introduced to her chemo nurse for the day. I tried not to stare, but I couldn't help but notice the looks on people's faces as we walked past; it was like a wax museum entirely dedicated to sadness, to intolerable suffering. Only it wasn't them who were on 'display,' it was us.

It was a bit like entering an unfamiliar pub for the first time and slowly becoming aware that, as you make your way to the end of the bar, you're the only person in the whole place who isn't a regular. As we made our way across the room their faces all twisted into the same expression that seemed to ask the same questions. *What is she doing here? What type of cancer could this beautiful young girl have? What's a nice girl like you doing in a place like this?*

But as soon as she walked into the room, you could also sense a change in the grim atmosphere. Erin's youth and outgoing personality lifted some of the gloom of the place. Erin began a number of friendly conversations and her smiling face opened a lot of closed eyes that day (and minds, for that matter).

The nurses had to access Erin's Port-A-Cath for the first time. It was a painful experience. If you don't know what a Porta-A-Cath is, or what one is used for, trust me, you don't want to know. Dr. Malik had surgically implanted a Port-A-Cath under Erin's skin, just below her right shoulder, which has a line attached that runs directly to her heart. The device is quite similar to an insulin cap that a diabetic would use to pull insulin through when they load a syringe. Approximately an inch or 2.5 cm in diameter, the Port-A-Cath can be used to draw blood out of the body in addition to administering chemo drugs into the body. It was designed to provide a convenience for the nurses and the patient, by eliminating the need to start an IV each time a patient requires treatment.

But for some reason, the nurses had a real problem each time they tried to draw some blood from the port. They tried three times, pushing a butterfly needle into the aperture, getting nothing but air. This was an indication that either the access itself wasn't working, or they hadn't accessed the port properly. Finally, one of the younger nurses had an idea. She decided Erin should reposition herself on the recliner. Next, they had Erin recline fully by lowering her head and elevating her legs. This seemed to work. The nurse's name was Karla, but we came to know her as "nurse Power." She was one of the younger and more energetic nurses in the chemo ward, and we always enjoyed one another's company. Karla started an infusion through Erin's Port-A-Cath with a saline IV for one hour and then followed up with her first round of drugs.

At about 2:00 p.m., we had our first visitor. Jan had decided to stop in, but didn't stay very long. I couldn't blame her. God knows we all wanted to turn right back around when we first walked in. We never verbally agreed on it, but I knew that Brett and I were going to be there each and every time Erin was scheduled for her treatments. It's something we always did. I think I missed one session because I had a terrible cold and didn't want to spread any germs. God only knows the patients' immune systems were probably destroyed and they already had enough on their plate without me contaminating the ward and giving them pneumonia.

It took the entire day to infuse the three drugs. They finally let us go around 4:30 p.m. As we were leaving, they gave us a handful of anti-nausea pills and some instructions on how to take them. The pills had a different name, but it was the same medication given to RoseMarie when she had her chemo. Basically, the next step was simply to *go home and expect to vomit your guts out!* This is what happens with almost all chemo patients.

One of the senior nurses gave us a very good explanation of why this happens. She told Erin that chemo is designed to kill any cells in the body that are dividing too quickly. But chemo is also non-selective: it kills the good cells along with the bad ones. However, it was expected that the normal cells would reproduce, while the cancer cells would hopefully be unable to repair themselves and eventually die off. Some of the fastest subdividing cells in the body are in the stomach, hair and skin, and this is why a person develops nausea, their hair falls out, or skin irritations and rashes occur.

According to the Native American Cancer Research Corporation, "there are more than fifty different chemotherapy drugs and the drugs are used in different proportions and combinations based on the specific cancer diagnostic information. In general, chemotherapy drugs affect the DNA of the cells by interfering with cell duplication. These drugs affect both the cancerous and the healthy cell DNA. The healthy cells that are particularly susceptible to chemotherapeutic drugs are those which multiply quickly, like the skin (including body, facial, and head hair) gastrointestinal tract, and bone marrow."[1]

---

1 Native American Cancer Research Corporation, http://natamcancer.org/page136.html. Accessed on June 1, 2014.

Oddly enough, this was the most positive and motivating thing that we had heard all day. It meant that each time Erin vomited we would know that no matter how awful she felt, the cancer would be getting it worse. Another image from the past flashed before me. I saw Dr. Hubbard telling RoseMarie that for strong cancer you needed strong medicine. *We're at war,* I thought, *and before now the enemy went about largely uncontested. No more. Now we launch a full-scale counter-offensive. Now we've got more than just a chance, we have a fighting chance.*

Brett and I accompanied Erin to all of her chemo treatments. One of us was always her shadow. Neither of us wished to God that Erin would have to be there, so there was no way we would ever let her go it alone. I think both Brett and I are proud of the fact to this day that Erin was never alone, that she always had one of us helping her through every treatment. Brett's mother, Lyn, always referred to Erin as "the daughter I never had." Lyn always sent a huge care package for Erin to help her get through those long days in the chemo chair. She packed everything from snacks to munch on to small puzzles and magazines to read, and every bag always had some small gift for Erin buried within it. Sometimes, I swear that bag weighed ten pounds. Brett always carried her "Lyn bag."

Brett used to tell us how his mom loved to shop. I only believe it was because she loved Erin. I have a special place in my heart for Brett. I am so proud of him. He said he would be there for Erin and he always was. Erin sure knew how to pick the good ones! Thank you very much Lyn for pounding the pavement. Brett always said "it gives Mom an excuse to shop."

It's unfortunate I never really got to know Brett personally before Erin got sick. I came to realize that my daughter had found a very special young man. He chose to be with her and stay with her because he loved her. I admire him for recognizing how special Erin was no matter what the cancer had destroyed. For Brett, nothing could take away the beautiful person Erin was.

Brett and I had one thing in common for sure: we both loved Erin. Brett was just another reason. I came to know I was the luckiest Dad in the world. I raised Erin for twenty years and watched her develop into a beautiful young lady.

Chapter Twelve

OUR FIGHT BEGINS

In early February, we received a phone call from a woman named Katherine Osczevski. Katherine is a genetic counselor with the Royal University Hospital in Saskatoon and was calling to confirm they received a referral from Dr. Malik concerning genetic testing and required Erin's consent to test her blood. The next day Erin signed the necessary paperwork to have her blood drawn. We made our way to the Pasqua Hospital yet again, where a requisition from Dr. Huntsman was waiting for us requesting 40cc (ml.) of blood for his team at the CTAG laboratory in Vancouver. Another 10cc was also to be drawn and sent to a Mt. Sinai clinical laboratory in California. Both were independent tests looking for a protein-truncating mutation in Erin's blood, the CDH1 gene. All in all, Erin had to have 14 vials of blood drawn. Erin hated needles, but she never complained about having to do it.

We continued with Erin's fifth chemo treatment session. Each treatment lasted about three weeks. Because of the cancer, Erin's stomach wasn't working properly and she required a supplemental food source for nourishment. Every night since the surgery, I had to give Erin a supplemental feeding of Jevity 1.2 through her J-Tube using a food pump. On February 21st, Erin had a referral to see a surgical oncologist in Calgary. Dr. Aboo had recommended Dr. Oliver Bathe at the Tom Baker Cancer Centre, a highly skilled surgeon and oncologist at the Foothills Hospital.

The night before Erin, Jared and I packed her food pump, IV pole and departed on WestJet's last flight of the day into Calgary. Because it was winter, it was already dark by the time we arrived around 9:00 in the evening. Erin and I looked out the window. The city lit up the night sky. All we could see from the air were lights. I had read somewhere that Calgary had just blossomed to one million, so coming from Regina was a bit like coming from a smaller city in Alberta.

After landing, I rented a van at the airport to accommodate Erin's IV pole and drove us to a motel. I sometimes have trouble finding an address in Regina never mind driving at night in a huge city like Calgary. Needless to say, it was a good thing we got some directions on how to get to the motel or we might not have gotten to bed before midnight. We stayed at the Best Western just south of the University of Calgary and right across the street from McMahon Stadium, home of the Canadian Football League's (CFL) Calgary Stampeders. It was just a few blocks from the Foothills Hospital and the Tom Baker Cancer Centre. By the time we finally settled into the stiff sheets and boxy pillows of the motel, we were exhausted and Erin was thoroughly worn out from the trip.

The next morning we checked out of our room and made our way to the Health Sciences Centre, Area 5B for our 9:00 a.m. appointment. We followed the signs and eventually made our way into a parkade. The Foothills complex is huge. It's as big as a university and has as many off premise buildings as any campus I've ever seen. Although finding the parkade was relatively easy, it was only just the beginning. The real challenge was to find the right building but, thankfully, we almost walked straight into the side of it after we parked the car.

The Health Sciences Centre was crawling with students. We followed the flow of traffic and found our way to an information desk that would tell us how we might find our way to Area 5B. It sounded like an airplane hangar, like Area 51. I half expected someone to say, 'we'd tell you, but then we'd have to kill you.' Miraculously, we didn't get lost making our way to the fifth floor, but as luck would have it our success was all for naught. As soon as we found Area 5B we were instructed to go right back where we came in on the main floor and register. After the paperwork had been completed, we used our newly acquired expertise and walked straight to Erin's appointment.

When we arrived, the office person gave Erin a questionnaire to fill out and we sat in a waiting area sectioned off by dull grey partitions. Before long, a nurse called Erin so she could take her temperature and record her weight. We sat in the waiting area again. We browsed listlessly through some magazines until Erin was called again and taken into Dr. Bathe's office.

Dr. Bathe walked into the room wearing black dress pants, a white shirt and a brown tie. We introduced ourselves and began to discuss our reasons for coming to Calgary. We were there because the Foothills Hospital performed total gastrectomies more routinely than the hospitals in Saskatchewan, and because we knew that Dr. Bathe specialized in tumours of the liver, pancreas and the upper GI tract.

Dr. Bathe had already been briefed on Erin's condition by Dr. Aboo in a letter and he had seen Erin's CT and MRI images. We asked him about the possibility of surgery after Erin had completed her chemo treatments. Dr. Bathe was initially very skeptical but Erin was very optimistic. She was determined that she was coming back to Calgary in six months for surgery. We discussed the disease and the type of surgery that would be required. A total gastrectomy, after chemo, was Dr. Bathe's recommendation. I had so many questions. How often is this type of surgery performed? Is the reconstruction of an artificial pouch in place of total removal of the stomach a better option? How many other people have had this procedure?

We then discussed something called "abdominal chemo." This procedure involved direct application of chemotherapy inside the abdomen. I was excited about this concept and thought it would be effective in helping Erin's diffused form of cancer. Our consultation lasted approximately an hour. When we left Dr. Bath's office we were under the distinct impression that he didn't believe we would be back in six months. I had this sense that he didn't think Erin would be alive in six months, let alone be eligible for surgery. I didn't want to ask which one it was. Dr. Bathe was not smiling when we left. But, I wasn't going to argue with the Assistant Professor of Surgery and Oncology. He knew what he was talking about and he knows a lot about cancer. Erin too didn't like what she was hearing. In a firm voice she told Dr. Bathe, "I will see you in six months."

Dr. Bathe said, "You sound very sure of yourself."

Erin said, "I am."

On February 25th, Erin and I began to look to alternative medicine. After chemo, Erin's immune system had considerably weakened. She was always tired and sometimes could hardly function at all, so anything we thought we could try, we did. We had heard of a product called "Goji Juice" that was supposed to neutralize alkalinity in the body and help give a person more energy. We purchased a couple of cases and Erin and I tried it. I didn't notice any immediate physical differences, but Erin said she felt that she had more energy.

Someone we knew mentioned a person in Regina who could get us in touch with a company called Mannatech Inc., a multinational firm that specializes in researching and developing products high in glyconutrients, the scientific name for plant carbohydrates or sugars. We figured nothing ventured, nothing gained, and Erin had everything to gain and nothing to lose. We thought it might be better for her overall health than chemo.

I called a representative of the company who introduced himself as Mr. Kazael. He invited us to meet with him and discuss the potential benefits of these herbal products. I never tried alternative medicine with Erin's mother and she passed away seven months after diagnosis. I wasn't going to ignore any possible hope Erin could find to strengthen her mental confidence. Mr. Kazael seemed to be a very honest and somewhat outspoken businessman. He introduced Erin and I to his wife and children and we became friends instantly. Erin and Mr. Kazael's wife, Nataline, seemed to have a great deal in common for two people who had never met before. It wasn't specific things, so much as the way their personalities seemed to perfectly and nearly instantaneously dovetail with one another. It was amazing to listen to them converse even only a few minutes after they first met.

We spent a long time with Mr. Kazael in his office that afternoon. I was hoping that, this time, things were happening for a reason, that our fortuitous encounter with Mr. Kazael had something to it that we could grasp. After meeting with Mr. Kazael, Erin decided to try it out. We went ahead and ordered a "starter kit" of Mannatech products called "Ambrotose," a blend of eight different sugars derived mainly from plants that were said to bolster the immune system. I know, dear reader, what you must be thinking: the whole thing reeks of snake oil. But remember that we called them, they never called us. You probably won't be surprised to hear that the Ambrotose wasn't cheap either. Obviously, I wasn't thinking about the money. The question was simply moot: I couldn't put a value on Erin's life, or her wellbeing. If Erin believed it could help her, I was completely in favour of the idea. I would have shot down the moon.

Katherine and the doctors at the Royal University Hospital in Saskatoon understood that Erin's deteriorating health would make travel difficult, so on March 17th, Jan, Brett and I accompanied Erin to the General Hospital in Regina for a teleconference with our genetic counsellor. Katherine explained that a certain percentage of people inherited the CDH1 mutation from either parent. She explained that cells carrying a "bad copy" of the gene can lose their programming and begin to multiply uncontrollably. "Cancer," she said, "is essentially a word for cells that have lost control."

CDH1 carriers already have one bad copy of their cells. As a result, they are at much higher risk of developing gastric cancer than someone in the general population. The odds were sobering. A person holds a 50/50 chance of inheriting the bad copy from a carrier parent. Males have a sixty-seven per cent lifetime chance of developing Hereditary Diffuse Gastric Cancer if he inherited the gene. Females fare even worse: women have an eighty-three per cent lifetime chance of developing HDGC, and a forty per cent lifetime chance of developing lobular breast cancer, if inheriting the gene. Desperate times called for desperate measures. After the genetic consultation, Erin was told again about the fact that there was not much that could be done.

The shit had hit the fan. Despite having seen a near army of doctors and medical professionals of some sort, this was the first time that someone had actually made a connection between RoseMarie's cancer and Erin's cancer. It only took 16 freaking years. Not only that, now they tell us that a blood test had been developed and in use since 2005 – *2005!* – to screen for the mutation. Oh, okay. I forgot that there was a catch – you actually have to have the disease before they can test anyone in your family for the mutation. They were only telling us this now, when everyone was telling us it was already too late.

Since 2005, there has been a test and nobody had told us the disease was hereditary. I knew the symptoms were all too similar, but I didn't know what it was called, where it had come from or what the connection was. All this time it seemed like a cruel twist of fate, like something out of the book of Job, the outcome of a stupid wager between capricious deities. A bad cosmic joke.

I'm sitting there in front of the monitor and I'm stewing. I felt something of the impotent rage that happens when you *just* miss something – like an elevator or a bus – multiplied one billion times. What Erin said next, I will never forget. It blew me right away. She smiled a little, looked at Katherine and said, "They may not be able to help me, but I may be able to help my family." For Erin it was never about Erin. It was only ever about what she could do for the rest of us.

In mid-March, we were told the initial results of Erin's blood screenings came back from the lab in Saskatoon, but they wouldn't be released until a second set of blood tests had been run. Dr. Huntsman's team was the first to find the CDH1 mutation. Dr. Huntsman holds an MD, FRCPC, FCCMG and is an Assistant Professor of Pathology at the University of British Columbia. He a genetic pathologist of Hereditary Cancer Programs at British Columbia Cancer Agency. They confirmed he had received Erin's blood on February 7, 2007. A week later, we received confirmation that the U.S. laboratory had also found a protein truncating mutation, a "2100deLT, in exon 13 of the CDH1 gene."

Thanks to Chief they found this mutation and other relatives can now be tested for CDH1. Unfortunately, they have to have an affected person before any DNA testing can be done. This opens up a whole new can of worms. We now know that the disease is hereditary and that any relatives on RoseMarie's side of the family tree could be a potential carrier. They won't even realize that they've inherited a killer gene.

Our calendar was gradually filling with medical appointments for both Erin and Jared and on top of everything else, it was beginning to look something like a blacked-out bingo card. Jared was now in Grade 12 and about to graduate. His hockey team had qualified for the provincial championship and he was working part-time for the Saskatchewan Hockey Association and Hockey Regina as a referee, while also working part-time at a grocery store. To make matters worse, Jared had recently broken his wrist while on a snowboarding trip.

Like the rest of us, Jared was just trying to live his life. While Erin was in the throes of her third session of chemo treatments, Jared was beginning medical testing for the possibility that he could have inherited the CDH1 mutation. The screening process would once again have to go through Saskatoon, and just as before, the whole process took a long time to coordinate. The inconveniences were nothing when one thought about the consequences. Erin had likely saved Jared's life.

Dr. Malik booked Jared for several gastric scopes until we could find out if he was a genetic carrier and we collectively held our breath: did Jared inherit the CDH1 mutation from his mother?

Erin, Brett and I had made an appointment to meet Dr. Aboo at his clinic. Erin's appetite and her ability to swallow had substantially improved since the previous chemo treatments. She was beginning to regain some weight, which came out to about 55 kilograms (120 pounds). Erin told Dr. Aboo that she had blurred vision for a few days after her last chemotherapy session, so Dr. Aboo scheduled a series of CT Scans and MRI's of the abdomen and pelvis to be taken after completion of the fourth round of chemotherapy. Erin was then going to be reassessed by Dr. Bathe to see whether or not she would be eligible for another surgery.

April 11, 2007. Brett and I always accompanied Erin to chemo, but this time Erin said I didn't have be there. I think she was trying to spare me something of the pain. But I said I was going anyway.

"Yes," I said, "you have no idea how badly I do have to be there, for every second of it."

Erin continued with her fourth round of chemo. Each time we came in, they weighed her and each time Erin had gained a little more weight; now she was up to around 57 kilograms. Amidst the gloom of everyday life under the auspices of the disease, this was cause for minor celebration. Indeed, every time Erin discovered that she had gained a little weight, she was overjoyed (not a very common thing among young women today, I imagine).

Erin had now been undergoing chemotherapy for three months. Dr. Aboo let us know he was going to be away for a few weeks, so he scheduled a couple of diagnostic scans to be completed before he returned and told us he had made arrangements for another oncologist to care for Erin in his absence.

But things continued heading south. The morning Erin was scheduled to have her abdominal CT scan (April 27th), she mentioned she was having sharp pains in her chest whenever she took a deep breath. I thought little of it at the time; if whatever it was, was significant, surely something would show up on the CT scan.

Shortly after we returned home from the hospital, Erin went out to visit her friend Nikki. While she was out, the Clinic called her cell phone and sure enough, we were to return immediately. It was almost 4:30 in the afternoon when we arrived. When we arrived, an oncologist was already waiting for us. In a thick South African accent, the oncologist told Erin that the CT had detected blood clots in both of her lungs and that she would have to have a heparin injection immediately to prevent any further clots from developing. Erin asked what would happen if she didn't take the injections right away. The doctor replied simply and directly, "You'll die."

The bluntness of the words stung. I asked why he was recommending heparin rather than warfarin, another anticoagulant. The oncologist told us that the heparin would act much more quickly, and could be easily reversed should any adverse effects occur. Warfarin, which is usually taken orally rather than through injection, is much slower acting and also more difficult to reverse. In moments, Erin was given her first injection. The oncologist wrote out a prescription for one injection a day for three days, then Erin would need to return to the hospital for a blood test.

The injections lasted about a week until Dr. Aboo returned. When he discovered what had happened, he wanted Erin to stop using the heparin, and prescribed warfarin instead. She was to take 1 to 2 milligrams of the small brown tablets a day until her blood levels were stable, but this was a very hard thing to control. Erin's blood levels varied from week to week and seemed to be affected by whatever she ate. When we asked Dr. Aboo what might be causing the blood clots in Erin's lungs, he simply stated that some people were susceptible to clotting while on chemo.

We asked how long Erin would have to remain on the blood thinner, and Dr. Aboo's answer wasn't encouraging: Erin would likely have to be on warfarin for the rest of her life. Depending on who you were, each person in the room had their own take on what that phrase – the rest of your life – might mean. To Erin, it may have sounded like a long time; the rest of a life barely begun.

I thought I heard something else. I heard the past banging in my ears like distant drums, the harbinger of some impending, unseen doom. I thought I saw it poised like a jungle cat in the darkness, the sinews of its muscles coiled, glinting in moonlight, ready to spring and destroy us all.

Chapter Thirteen

AMAZING PEOPLE

"It's not the years in your life
but the life in your years that count."
—Adlai E. Stevenson

Before she became ill, Erin was working part-time for a Co-op grocery store in north Regina. She had worked part-time throughout high school and continued on when she began attending university. Knowing Erin, I'm sure that when she told her friends and co-workers she had cancer and needed surgery right away, she probably didn't make too big of a deal about it or let them know exactly how serious things were.

One day I received a phone call from Pam, one of Erin's fellow employees at the Co-op. She asked how Erin was doing and then told me they were planning a couple of fundraisers to show their support: a "Steak Night" and a "Walk-a-thon." Pam said everyone in the store felt Erin's absence, that they missed seeing her smiling face at Customer Service. Erin had already let the store know she would have to return to Calgary in six months after completing chemo to have a total gastrectomy. Erin's steak night was to be held on April 28th. The "Walk-for-Erin," which was to take place in the large park in the heart of the city, was scheduled for the next day.

In May 2007, Erin began her fifth session of chemo. Many of the nurses around the chemo ward had now become familiar and friendly faces. As I've said before, the mood of the place always seemed to change whenever Erin walked in. I'm not sure if it was her youth, her positive attitude, or her overall personality, but Erin always radiated a certain cheeriness that seemed to make the whole atmosphere vibrate on a different wavelength. It was always something of a marvel. I was never really sure how she managed it. Heck, I couldn't even manage it, and I wasn't even the sick one.

For the past two months, Erin had been complaining about some discomfort in her tailbone, so Dr. Aboo put in a request for Erin to go to the General Hospital for a bone scan. We received the results a few days later and everything appeared to be normal. Finally some good news, we thought, finally something to be thankful for. But such news couldn't be called authentically 'good,' not really. It was simply the absence of bad news. I pondered this. Is health the mere absence of sickness? The consequences of such an idea seem dire. As the poet W.B. Yeats once wrote, "Things fall apart; the centre cannot hold."

Health would no longer be anything real, nothing substantive, a kind of illusion that we simply *needed* in order to convince ourselves things are normal, that the world makes sense. Without it we would be constantly overwhelmed, swept away in a great flux of suffering. It would mean that we could no longer think of the disease as a deviation from the norm; rather, health would become the anomaly, the absolute gift. Life is fragility itself.

A few weeks later, Jan and I drove Jared to Saskatoon for a genetic consultation with Katherine. It would be the first time we met Katherine face to face, rather than speaking to her through a monitor. I couldn't believe we had to do this again. Katherine reiterated the percentages of inheriting the CDH1 mutation from either parent. She described to Jared how cells carrying the bad copy of the gene can lose their programming and begin multiplying uncontrollably (things fall apart, the centre does not hold). Carriers of the mutation already had one bad copy in all their cells. As a result, they would be at a much higher risk of developing gastric cancer than someone in the general population. I already knew all of this, but Jared had to hear it for himself. Two things in particular were important where Jared was concerned: A person had a 50/50 chance of inheriting the bad copy from a carrier parent. Once inherited, a male had a sixty-seven per cent lifetime chance of developing HDGC.

Just as with Erin, Katherine scheduled a round of blood tests for Jared, and we waited to see whether lightning struck thrice. But by June, we still hadn't heard anything. Dr. Aboo was still waiting for test results from Calgary concerning Erin's chances for surgery. He didn't want Erin to discontinue chemotherapy until he could coordinate the end of the treatment with a potential surgery date. In the meantime, Erin would begin her sixth round of chemo treatments.

Throughout the entire process, Erin's friends kept the home fires burning. A number of them got together and decided to organize a team for the 2007 Cancer Relay for Life. Brett and some of Erin's guy friends put their respective talents together and began engineering plans to build a float. They decided they were all going to dress up as pirates and their float would be a great big pirate ship.

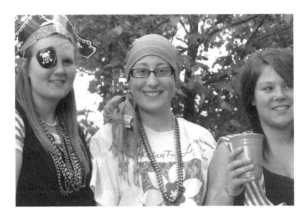

Lindsay, Erin, Lisa

The float had to be constructed in such a manner that it would be strong enough to carry the weight of just one person: Erin, their ship's captain. The float had to be portable, large enough for the team to push but also light enough to be carried. They did an amazing job. The ship looked great and Erin's friends placed second overall in raising the most money for the Canadian Cancer Society by an individual team: a total of $8,930.15. They accomplished this by holding a variety of fundraising events in the weeks prior to the Relay itself: everything from a car wash in a Walmart parking lot to selling specially made orange I ♥ ERIN wristbands. The wristbands were the brainchild of Erin's friend Lindsay. She knew that orange was my favorite colour and that Erin was my favourite, my *only*, daughter. I remember the Relay For Life as if it happened yesterday. Erin and I walked around the track several times with several different people and shared the day with hundreds of other cancer survivors.

Despite the mostly jubilant and hopeful atmosphere, Erin wasn't feeling great. She had been having severe migraine headaches for the past few days and that day wasn't any different. But Erin never complained. She put on a brave face when her friends were around and tried to appear as though everything was fine. That was just her nature; only her family would know the extent of her pain.

The pictures we took at the Relay tell the whole story. You can see pain in my daughter's eyes. You can see that she was trying to do the impossible; she was trying to make the camera lie. Erin, Jan and I spent the entire event surrounded by Erin's extraordinary friends. Jared would show up later in the evening for the candlelight vigil that closes out the Relay every year in honour of those that lost their fight.

We found RoseMarie's name among the three thousand plus decorated luminaria lining the walkway of the park. Erin's friends had created their own luminaria in honour of their ship's "captain," placing it right next to RoseMarie's. Under Erin's name, illuminated in bright green paint, her friends had written *"Our Hero."*

Erin wanted to stay and celebrate the entire twenty-four hour event with her friends, but the pain was too much and we had to take her home. Erin had told me that this had always bothered her. She was beginning to feel disconnected, isolated, like the disease was sweeping her away from life.

It was now mid-June and we were still waiting for a surgeon from Calgary to get in contact with us. When we last visited Dr. Bathe, he wasn't at all certain that Erin would be back for surgery, but Erin was determined. There had been setbacks, to be sure – the blood clots back in April and the persisting migraines – but Erin was eating well, well enough to hold her normal weight.

However, the migraines were fast becoming unbearable in their severity and tenacity, occurring in shorter and shorter intervals and lasting for longer periods of time. When we let Dr. Aboo know that the migraines were getting worse, he made immediate arrangements for Erin to see a neurologist. I told Erin I wanted her to sleep upstairs so I could keep a close eye on her condition. We had tried just about everything in the medicine cabinet to help with Erin's migraines. Two extra-strength Tylenol temporarily did the job, and Erin was finally able to get a little bit of sleep.

She had only slept about four hours before the next attack, which continued on and off until we arrived at the neurologist's office the next morning. Even while we were sitting in the waiting room, Erin had another vicious migraine. The receptionist noticed Erin was in a great deal of discomfort and let the neurologist know right away of her condition. We were immediately called into the office and asked the usual questions concerning family history. The doctor then performed a series of tendon reflex tests, checking Erin's neck, pupils, and extraocular movements. After these preliminaries, the neurologist said he believed Erin's migraines and her nausea had been triggered by the chemo. In his view, there was only a five per cent chance that the headaches could be linked to the disease. I liked to think there was a ninety-five per cent chance *that it wasn't*.

We followed the doctor downstairs to the Emergency Room where he gave Erin hits of Demerol and Gravol to help relieve the headaches and wrote out a prescription for 10 milligrams of Maxalt RPD, a medication designed to relieve headaches by constricting the dilated blood vessels inside the head that cause migraines.

There was still the possibility that the headaches were symptoms of meningitis, but there was no way to be sure without doing a spinal tap. This didn't sound like fun. Erin and I had never heard of this procedure before. The only Spinal Tap I knew about was that fake metal band from the eighties. When I got to know the real thing, it suddenly seemed less funny. The term speaks for itself: the doctors freeze an area in the lower back and very carefully put a *very large* needle into the spinal cord to withdraw three or four vials of cerebrospinal fluid. However, the neurologist said it wasn't safe to do a spinal tap yet because Erin was still on blood thinners.

We returned home but after a few hours it was certain that the Maxalt wasn't helping. I called Dr. Aboo early the next morning and told him about the persistence of Erin's migraines and that I couldn't find any alternatives that would effectively block out the pain. Pumping Erin full of Tylenol 3's temporarily caused the pain to subside, but not a few hours would go by before the headaches would return in full force.

Dr. Aboo wrote Erin a new prescription and told me I would have to pick it up at the Allan Blair Cancer Centre. After I got to the Centre and picked up the new prescription, I then drove to the pharmacy. We had made so many trips to this particular pharmacy to fill out Erin's multiple prescriptions that I had come to know many of the pharmacists by their first names.

On this particular day a pharmacist by the name of Bev was working. Bev examined the crumpled bit of paper with Dr. Aboo's inked scrawl, scrunching her forehead. After a few moments she said they couldn't possibly fill out the prescription. Confused, I asked her why. Bev went on to say that they neither handle nor stock this particular drug. Still confused, I asked what it was.

"Well!" Bev said, "It's marijuana. The prescription is in pill form but, yeah, it's marijuana!"

I was surprised to say the least. I wondered whether or not my luck might be better served behind the portables of a high school. Bev just shrugged and said that the only pharmacy that could fill this type of prescription was the Allan Blair itself. I had something of a *"duh"* moment that made me feel like I was the one smoking up. *So that's what Dr. Aboo meant when he said I had to pick it up at the Clinic.* I returned to the Centre that day and finally managed to fill out Erin's prescription.

However, when it came time to actually give Erin her first pill, I started having second thoughts. Rather than give Erin the marijuana right away, I decided I would go back to see Bev at our regular pharmacy and see if there was anything else available for severe migraines. Bev said some people had found Tylenol Ultra worked. I figured I had nothing to lose but the expense. I was just hoping it would do something to help Erin.

Unfortunately, we soon discovered that even the Tylenol Ultra's did very little. On top of this, Erin was no longer eating very well. Just like with RoseMarie, Erin's stomach was quickly becoming incapable of digesting almost anything, save water and the horde of prescription medications that were supposed to be taken orally. By early afternoon of the next day I was nearly out of ideas. The only option left was to try the marijuana capsules. I discussed it with Erin and she agreed to give it a try. I gave her a single capsule with a glass of water and waited to see if it would stay down.

Through trial and error we had discovered which medications Erin could take orally without vomiting. This time was no different, Erin vomited shortly after taking her first capsule. I wasn't sure if the pill had been down long enough to have been absorbed into her system, so we decided to try another capsule in a few hours, just to be on the safe side.

After about twenty minutes, however, Erin began having hallucinations. She began staring at her hands, telling me they looked funny and felt strange. Her breathing became short and sporadic and soon her eyes began rolling around crazily in their sockets. A splash of translucent spittle pooled and descended in thick ropes from the side of her mouth. I was terrified. Brett and I immediately tried to get Erin to stand upright, but she passed out the moment she was vertical. Erin fell limp in our arms with the weight of a dead thing, collapsed like a marionette whose strings have gone completely slack in the absence of the puppeteer's hands.

As the two of us struggled to move her, Erin suddenly came to and vomited. I began to panic. All I could remember from my CPR courses years ago was that if a person was believed to be unconscious, they could choke on their vomit and you had to clear an airway to prevent them from swallowing their tongue. Erin's head was lolling from side to side. Using my index and middle fingers I tried to pull Erin's tongue to the front of her mouth to prevent her from choking. Big mistake.

Erin began to seizure and her jaw clamped down like a bear trap, nearly taking my fingers clean off. She began making growling noises that sounded like a cornered animal. With Brett's help, I managed to pry open Erin's jaw.

I left her with Brett and quickly ran next door. Our neighbours, fortunately for us, were both paramedics. We ran back to the house and they helped us stabilize Erin until an ambulance arrived.

The EMT's were kind enough to allow me to ride in the back of the ambulance so I could stay with Erin until we arrived at the hospital. Thankfully, the seizures eased up en route. Erin gradually regained consciousness and managed to successfully respond to the paramedic's questions about what she remembered about what had happened, what her name was, how she was feeling.

Erin smiled weakly when I said, "Welcome back, Chief." I felt like I had aged ten years since I last heard her voice.

When we arrived at the Emergency Department the nurses were quick to give Erin the medical attention she needed. We were in for a very long night. Erin had never had a seizure before. The ER doctor requested another CT scan; this would be Erin's third CT in about a week. As fate would have it, Dr. Malik walked by while we were waiting for Erin to be taken to Radiology. I asked him what he was doing there so late and he told us he was on call. But he seemed even more surprised to see us than we were to see him. I told him about Erin's seizure after having taken the marijuana pills and asked if it would be possible that Erin could have had an allergic reaction.

The situation was bizarre. Dr. Malik was fairly certain the marijuana wouldn't have likely caused the seizure; if anything, it should have prevented it. Erin's CT scan came back negative, yet she continued having severe migraines, even while in the hospital. The nurses started an IV and tried a couple of different medications to control the attacks. Nobody could figure out exactly why the seizure had happened. What they did know was that the marijuana probably had nothing to do with it.

Erin was to stay overnight for observation. Different doctors tried different ways of controlling Erin's headaches, but by the end of the night all remained baffled as to what had caused her seizure. As always, I stayed with her. The nurses rolled in an old recliner chair so I could sit beside Erin during the night. It wasn't comfortable. The vinyl stuck to the sweat on my arms and legs and the reclining mechanism seemed to be broken. Of course, it isn't fair to complain. That large illuminated "H" near the roof of the building doesn't stand for hotel.

The next day, the ER doctor wanted to check Erin's spinal fluid and asked permission to do a spinal tap. Permissions were a mere formality, at this point Erin really had no choice. The migraines had become so severe that the doctors suspected spinal meningitis. They wheeled Erin's bed into a different room where they had everything already set up. I waited outside the procedure room until they were finished. There are risks in everything we do in life, but pushing a needle into someone's spinal cord sounded pretty risky to me.

After the procedure was finished the doctor told me that when he tapped Erin's spinal cord the fluid that came out wasn't clear, as it was supposed to be. This wasn't a good sign. Although a clear sample didn't altogether rule out the possibility of viral meningitis, the fluid that came out of Erin's spinal cord was yellowish and viscous. A sample was sent off to the Cytology Lab. Until the results were back, Erin was to be placed under quarantine.

Chapter Fourteen

WARD 3B

"We must embrace pain and burn it as a fuel for our journey."
—*Kenji Miyazawa*

The longer we spent in the Emergency Department the more anxious I became. Emergency was the last place in the hospital that a cancer patient should spend more than twenty-four hours. Chemo had practically annihilated Erin's immune system, leaving her vulnerable to the potentially noxious mixture of bugs floating about the intersections of the Emergency Room. To make matters worse, the doctors now suspected Erin of having spinal meningitis. We would have to be sequestered in an isolation room in the Emergency Room until a hospital bed could be found. This was unacceptable.

I walked out of the Emergency Department, down the hall, and straight to the Allan Blair Cancer Centre. I wasn't happy to say the least. I went to have a chat, *mano a mano*, with Erin's oncologist. The receptionist asked if I had an appointment or if Dr. Aboo was expecting me. I told her that I didn't, but to please tell him that is was very important that I see him right away. She contacted him immediately and told me that Dr. Aboo would be right out. As we spoke, I realized he wasn't at all aware that Erin was in Emergency. He could tell from my voice I desperately wanted Erin to be moved out of there as soon as possible. Dr. Aboo called the Emergency Department and had Erin discharged.

She was to be admitted to 3B, the Cancer Ward. When we arrived, Erin was moved into a private isolation room. As a precautionary measure, everyone entering the room had to wear a full-length yellow hospital gown, gloves and a mask. It didn't matter. I decided right then that my place was

93

going to be with Erin. I wasn't going home any more. I couldn't leave her alone, isolated. The next day, Erin began complaining about blurred vision. At times, she said that she was even having multiple vision. She also began to notice a tingling sensation in one hand. Sometimes her legs went numb. We mentioned this to the nurses, thinking these might be symptoms associated with the meningitis. Erin's spinal tap results weren't back yet, but Erin's symptoms were so pronounced that Dr. Aboo started treating her for meningitis immediately. She began taking large amounts of antibiotics intravenously. I took up permanent residence in another hospital recliner that was part of the furniture in her room.

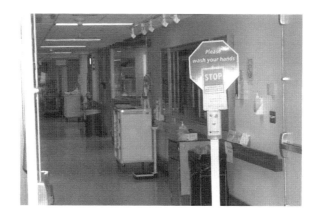

Things improved enough that Erin and I managed to convince the doctors she would be well enough to go home on a two-day pass the following weekend. It would be a chance for Erin to see both her family and friends without everyone having to be quarantined from one another. There was also Jared's Grade 12 Cap & Gown Graduation Ceremonies. It was great to see Erin dressed up and there for Jared on his special day. I know he was proud to see his sister there. Although Erin didn't say a word, I could tell the two-hour long ceremony had completely exhausted her. We all attended Jared's Graduation Banquet Dinner, along with Erin and Jared's grandparents.

But, shortly after arriving at the hall, Erin began to feel nauseous and weak. We weren't taking any chances, and I immediately began to make plans to have someone take Erin to the hospital while I went home to change. That was the plan. But Erin changed all that.

"This is Jared's big night, Dad. He needs you to be here. I'll get a ride to the hospital with Brett and Lyn. Don't worry, I'll be ok. You can come back up to the hospital later tonight. I'll be fine, don't worry."

Erin was right and, under the circumstances, I couldn't be in both places at once. She couldn't be there, so she wanted me to stay. She always set an example by thinking of others before thinking of herself. That night, Erin reminded me I had to share myself and some of my time with Jared. Sometimes you can't control what happens. I didn't know what would happen to Erin that night, but Erin made me realize that Jared needed me just as much as she did.

Between the maelstroms and monotonies that had taken over our lives since the diagnosis of Erin's illness, Jared was still growing up, and he was still my son. I reluctantly agreed and watched Lyn take Erin to the hospital. It was twilight and the streetlights were just flickering on as I made my way back inside the banquet hall. Shortly after the dance began, I left the convention centre to go to the hospital. When I arrived, Erin looked better and was sleeping comfortably. For once, a night passed without incident.

Chapter Fifteen

WHY ME?

"He who has health, has hope.
And he who has hope, has everything."
—Thomas Carlyle

June 26th was Erin's grandma's birthday, but we would be too busy to celebrate. We were out again on a day pass, but we weren't really going anywhere. Over the past few months, Erin had begun to develop small red lesions over her body. Our weekend pass turned into an arranged visit to a skin specialist. We were hoping this was yet another symptom of the chemo. Erin had more biopsies taken and a specimen was sent for a culture, fungal bacterial infections and cytology. Again, we awaited the results.

The next day, Erin began to have severe pain and weakness in her legs whenever she tried to walk. A feeling of desperation gripped me, hard. The symptoms just kept mounting. While we were waiting for the results of one test to return, something else would happen that would necessitate a different test, and after we had taken *that* test, another symptom would unexpectedly crop up, and on and on.

I started thinking about alternative approaches and asked Dr. Aboo if we might try something like hypnosis. He looked surprised, but after a moment's pause he said, "Sure, why not?" I reassured him that this wouldn't be anything that he would be liable or responsible for, that it was my idea and if Erin was willing to give it a try, we would try. I figured that she had endured enough already.

I was really just hoping that hypnosis might help to block out the incessant pain, that it might provide a gentler alternative than continuously ravaging Erin's immune system with drugs. Nothing ventured, nothing gained, and Erin had nothing to lose and everything to gain.

The hypnotherapist agreed to visit us in the hospital, as Erin was too sick to travel by anything but ambulance. The therapist herself was a cancer survivor who had taught herself hypnosis and believed that she had been able to force the disease into remission. After a couple of sessions, it seemed as though Erin was walking a little better and without as much pain. But, like everything else we had tried beyond conventional medicine, the benefits were temporary, and things were just beginning to get real bad.

Erin's health was deteriorating rapidly. She continued to get weaker and weaker. Gradually, she began losing the use of her left arm. Her sight and her hearing were also getting worse. Whatever lucky stars Erin had on her side (if she had any at all) were burning out, one by one. We were about to find out just to what extent Murphy's Law had utterly taken over our lives when I got my first look at the Family Room in Ward 3B.

One afternoon, one of the social workers from the Allan Blair Cancer Centre and Dr. Salim – who was taking care of Erin while Dr. Aboo was away at a conference – escorted me into a private room with a pull-out bed, small lamp, and recliner. The room smelled faintly the way plastic flowers smell when they're trying too hard to smell like real flowers.

The staff closed the door and asked me to have a seat. Dr. Salim had the difficult task of telling me that Erin's disease had metastasized. I had heard Dr. Aboo use the term before, but I never really knew exactly what it meant. From the grave look on Dr. Salim's face, I knew that it wasn't a good thing. It was about to get much worse than I could have ever anticipated.

"Erin doesn't have spinal meningitis," Dr. Salim said. "The cancer has spread into her spinal cord, and likely to her brain. The cancer is causing the migraines and the seizures."

Metastasis meant that the cancer cells had broken away from the primary tumour, entered Erin's bloodstream, and surreptitiously deposited themselves in otherwise healthy tissues elsewhere in the body, causing several malignant growths to develop in her brain. It also meant that we had no options left. When a cancer metastasizes, chances of survival plummet. The disease had begun to deploy its most final, fatal strategy, penetrating the very command centre of the body. The only thing left was surrender. Dr. Salim recommended that Erin be transferred to Palliative Care. They expected me to go back to Erin's room and tell her that there wasn't any hope, that the fight was over.

I could not do this. I remembered Erin telling me that one should never tell someone they only have a short time to live because it wasn't anyone's decision whether someone lived or died, it was up to God. I wasn't going to tell my only daughter that she was dying, that all her struggle would amount to nothing.

I felt like a cornered animal. It was the middle of the day but it seemed like shadows were everywhere before me, crowding the room. Dr. Salim and the social worker seemed to evaporate. All I could see of them were pale masks, Death in loose disguise. I begged them to continue Erin's treatment. I said that I simply wasn't going to take no for an answer. Erin and I weren't giving up. We weren't going to abandon the fight. I was her father and I was going to do everything possible to help my daughter. I would do anything not to face the reality of it. I would not go gently into that good night.

I begged them not to take hope away from my daughter, even when the disease had taken everything else. I asked them if they had any children, and what they would do if they were in my position. Dr. Salim's eyes brimmed with compassionate tears. He nodded his head and agreed to continue treatment. There would be no transfer to Palliative Care. I felt that I had to protect Erin from the truth. At the same time, I had never lied to Erin before, and if I was going to start then and there, the lie would have to be complete, absolute. It would have to be as complete and as absolute as truth itself.

I began to construct a grand illusion worthy of *"Life is Beautiful."* In that film, a Jewish-Italian father (played by Roberto Benigni) uses his imagination to shield his small son from the horrifying reality of their imprisonment in a concentration camp. Of course, I am by no means comparing the hospital to a concentration camp, but like Benigni's character, I wanted nothing more than to protect my daughter from the horrible realities of the disease. I began by making things perfectly clear with the doctors, the nurses, orderlies, porters, right down to the cleaning staff that *nobody* was to speak with Erin about the terminal nature of her condition, or leave her with any impression that she was untreatable.

Dr. Salim had informed Dr. Bathe that Erin would not be going to Calgary for any further testing or surgeries. Further treatment would likely involve another series of spinal taps, except that this time they would be injecting the chemo drugs directly into the base of Erin's spine. Erin didn't know everything, but she did know that the disease was now at Stage 4 and that her mother passed away from the same type of cancer. The only thing Erin knew that no one else could know was how much worse she was feeling.

After leaving the Family Room, I made my way back to Erin's room. I told her that her skin lesions were not byproducts of the chemo, but another manifestation of the cancer. I let her know that the disease had metastasized from her stomach and that it had spread to her spinal cord. When I told her of the painful course of treatment she would have to follow, her only response was, "You do what you have to do."

I thought I had made the right decision for Erin because I was doing what was right by her standards. She wasn't surrendering, we weren't giving up. She was in for the fight of her life, for her life. Maybe a glimmer of hope would prevail.

Treatment had to begin immediately, but things got even more complicated. We learned that the Saskatchewan Cancer Agency was possibly about to go on strike, which would affect the hospital pharmacy and anyone receiving chemotherapy. In the likelihood of a strike, Dr. Salim wanted Erin to have at least two rounds of treatment. When the time came for the first spinal tap, I helped Erin by kneeling in front of her holding her shoulders as she leaned her head forward against mine. Dr. Salim locally froze the area before pushing a large needle into Erin's lower back, perforating her spinal cord, and withdrawing a large amount of spinal fluid. He then replaced the same volume of extracted fluid with chemo drugs. Next, Erin was instructed to lie flat on her back for at least thirty minutes without moving or sitting up.

The treatment itself seemed grotesque, just as likely to kill as the disease itself. One thing was for certain, however, the disease would certainly kill. One could only hope that this new series of treatments were going to help by providing a certain *quality of time,* and with a little luck, and a lot of prayer, the disease would be forced into remission.

The next day Erin had another seizure. This time it was in the hospital and help was thankfully only a few steps away. Jan was helping Erin to the washroom. She needed help because the disease had, by this time, all but robbed Erin of her ability to walk. While they were returning to the bed, Erin told Jan that she felt really dizzy. Jan asked a nurse who happened to be in Erin's room at the time if she could help her get Erin into bed when suddenly Erin collapsed, pulling Jan, the nurse, and her IV pole to the floor in a heap.

I was waiting just outside of the room when I heard Jan frantically yelling for help. A nurse in the hall immediately paged for an ICU doctor and for Dr. Salim to come to the ward right away. Just as with Erin's prior collapses, I was scared shitless. Every time Erin went down, it was just like the first time. There was no getting used to it. An absolute terror seized every fibre of my being, the whole world spun off its axis, everything thrown off balance. The only thing that changed was the worry, the sick anxiety that accumulated in my soul. I was worried about Erin's condition and how fast it was deteriorating. There were so many medical personnel in Erin's room so quickly they could hardly get in and out of the door.

The next day, Dr. Salim decided that it was no longer safe to treat Erin through spinal taps, and that she would instead need something called an "Ommaya reservoir." Using the same spinal port over and over again gradually increased the risk of infection, and the Ommaya reservoir would allow the doctors to directly inject the chemo drugs into the cerebrospinal fluid through a port implanted in Erin's skull. If the spinal tap seemed grotesque, this sounded too awful to imagine, but we were nonetheless hopeful that something good would come out of it. The dice were warm and all we needed to do was throw…

Early on the morning of July 5, 2007, Erin was driven by ambulance from the Pasqua Hospital to the General Hospital to have the Ommaya reservoir surgically placed in her skull. The whole procedure was supposed to take approximately two hours. Tension and emotions were so high that Jan and I sat on opposite sides of the waiting room. I felt myself going crazy, waiting, watching the clock. Two hours passed and we hadn't heard anything. It was just before noon when they brought Erin out of the Operating Room. We were told that, despite the delay, the surgery had gone relatively well and that Erin would be moved back to the Pasqua Hospital after spending some time in the General's recovery room. As before, I was fortunate enough to be allowed to ride in the ambulance with Erin when it was time to return to the Pasqua Hospital.

When we arrived back at the ward, all of the nurses were anxious to see Erin. This wasn't the surgery Erin and I were hoping to get when all this started, but it seemed necessary at the time. It would save Erin the discomfort of having further spinal taps and would hopefully provide a safer, more effective means of treatment. Dr. Aboo was back from his conference. He wasn't pleased to discover that Erin's health had taken a turn for the worse while he had been away.

A few days later, Dr. Aboo arrived to give Erin her first session of chemotherapy through the Ommaya reservoir. When he tried to draw fluid, however, all that came back was blood. Something was wrong with the positioning of the reservoir's port, causing some consternation as to the ugly sounding possibility of intracranial bleeding. The neurosurgeon who had placed the reservoir was called in to confirm its position, and once again I was escorted into 3B's Family Room.

Emotions were running high again and I didn't want there to be a stand-off, so I told the social worker that I would ask for her help if I needed it. Jan had arrived in the interim and was with me when Dr.Aboo returned, the bearer of more bad news. He had consulted with his colleagues and the consensus was that Erin's condition was irreversible. She would likely only survive for a matter of days, weeks, at best.

It was the kind of news you expect from the very beginning but want to forget, something that sits there gnawing in the pit of the stomach, a formless indigestible mass, the place inside in which everything you never want to hear or believe sleeps and waits. They said we were going to lose Erin.

I said that I wasn't going to give up. I wouldn't let them take our hope away. I implored Dr. Aboo to refer Erin for more treatment. I told him that under no circumstances was Erin to be transferred to Palliative Care. Dr. Aboo finally conceded that there was one last possible treatment available: radiation. It would likely do more harm than good. I didn't care, we were going to fight until every last option had been exhausted.

★ ★ ★

That evening the **CFL**'s Saskatchewan Roughriders were playing their divisional rivals the Calgary Stampeders. The game was supposed to be blacked out locally, but it sold out, so the game aired on national television. As a series of network cameras panned across the sea of green and white Rider fans, a group of seemingly incongruous signs were printed by a few of Erin's friends, with the phrase "I love Erin" that stood out of the crowd.

The Riders won 49 to 8.

★ ★ ★

The oncologist responsible for Erin's radiation treatments paid us a visit the next afternoon. After asking Erin some questions and doing some preliminary examinations, the oncologist and I met outside of the room to discuss Erin's condition. She was *very* reluctant to offer Erin radiation therapy, and her professional opinion was that it wouldn't help things. She looked at me straight and said she had decided she wasn't going to approve the therapy. My face paled and I felt her gaze go through me as if I were a ghost. I asked her the same question I had already asked Dr. Aboo, "If it was your daughter, what would you do? Would you do nothing?"

She looked at me closely. I was shaking with sadness and anger. Finally, she agreed to set up a treatment program. Erin was scheduled for a total of five sessions over the next eight days, July 10th to 18th.

Of all the horrible things Erin had gone through, the radiation treatments were the worst. I was glad that Brett was usually along. Erin seemed to glow like a 100-watt bulb whenever he came to visit. He gave her strength that was otherwise being drained. I'm not sure I even want to describe what Erin had to go through. A feeling of guilt pressed upon me that went beyond measure. As a father, I've always tried to protect my daughter from harm. If that's what a father does, if that's our version of the Hippocratic Oath, then I'd gone completely the other way. I was now putting my daughter into a giant microwave oven and watching them nuke her brain.

The only way to put things into perspective is to understand why. Like some of the chemo treatments Erin had already experienced, cranial radiation is non-selective, meaning that it destroys both cancerous and normal cells without discrimination. Normal brain cells are expected to reproduce themselves while the cancer cells would be destroyed outright. I explained this to Erin and hoped the treatments did just that. But the oncologist was right. As we were about to find out, it was going to do more harm than good.

After the first day of Erin's treatment, we received word from the Genetics Lab at the Royal University Hospital in Saskatoon that Jared's test results were back. Due to circumstances with Erin, I decided we would postpone our trip. I told them that we would have to get in touch with Katherine at a later date. All of us sat suspended at the lip of a void.

Chapter Sixteen

A SPECIAL FRIENDSHIP

"Don't lose hope. When the sun goes down, the stars come out."
—*Unknown*

In the final week of July, I received a call from Pam, one of Erin's friends and co-workers at the Co-op. She said she knew someone who had contacts within the Saskatchewan Roughriders and that they could arrange for a player to come up to the hospital for a visit. I thought this was a fantastic idea and that we should keep it a surprise.

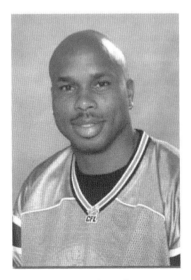

Kerry Joseph

On the afternoon of July 27th, Erin got one of the biggest (happiest) surprises of her life. That day Erin was very ill. She was trying to rest and was lying on her side, facing away from the doorway of the hospital room. I lightly touched Erin's shoulder to wake her up and told her she has a very special visitor today. Kerry Joseph, the Riders' quarterback, was here to see her. As she sleepily mumbled, "Yeah right, Dad" in that beautiful way young people do, I motioned for Mr. Joseph to approach the bed so that Erin could see him.

He walked up right behind her and said in a deep voice, "Hello, Erin."

You should have seen the expression on Erin's face ("surprise" doesn't cover it, by the way). Her eyes got very wide and in a small voice said, "Uh, hi."

If you know anything about Erin's personality by now, then you know that the whole time "KJ" was there, she never once talked about herself. It was all about football. Mr. Joseph brought out some autographed memorabilia and presented them to Erin.

Before he left, Erin asked him for a favour. "Can you pound the Edmonton Eskimos for me?"

Mr. Joseph had a big grin on his face and said, "Yeah, I can do that."

Before he left the hospital, I stepped out and thanked him for taking time out of his busy schedule to visit my daughter. I told him that Erin was only expected to live a very short time. She and a friend had been planning to go to all the Riders' home games that season, but Erin had been so sick she had not been able to attend a single game. Physically, Mr. Joseph is a big man. I came to realize his heart is just as big. I could see tears in his eyes when we shook hands and said our goodbyes.

The next day, we all gathered together to listen to the game in Erin's room. We had the radio tuned in and were listening to the local broadcast. We could see Mosaic Stadium in the near distance from Erin's room, and we could hear the dull roar of the crowd on big plays. The Riders were playing host to the Edmonton Eskimos.

The local station CKRM was doing colour commentary and we were surprised to hear Erin's name mentioned several times throughout the broadcast: the commentators kept talking about how Kerry Joseph wanted to dedicate the game to "a young lady who is very ill and battling cancer." Joseph went on to score the Riders' first rushing touchdown of the game, and in the background you could hear the sharp rise of the crowd, celebrating. Sure enough, Joseph and the Riders went on to beat the Eskimos 54–14, a promise he kept for Erin.

We were speechless. Most of the nurses knew that Joseph had been up to the ward the day before, and everyone was excited. I was later told that at half time Joseph approached his teammates and mentioned that he had been to the hospital to visit a young twenty-year-old Riders fan who was fighting for her life. All that she had asked was for the Riders to pound the Eskimos. The defence stood up and rallied around Erin's request. The score pretty much tells the rest of the story on that day.

The next day, Mr. Joseph came back to the hospital with his friend and teammate Yo Murphy, to present Erin with the game ball. We were definitely surprised; this time Joseph had shown up on his own accord. I could see he was fascinated by Erin's character. Like most people who had met Erin, Joseph seemed to find her personality infectious. After introducing Murphy, Erin had a strange expression on her face. "Is 'Yo' your real first name? Like, really?"

He laughed and said he was asked that question quite a lot. After visiting for a short time, Erin had one more favour to ask, "Would you please destroy the BC Lions for me?"

Kerry smiled and said, "You got it, kid."

Both players gave Erin a hug. Just before Joseph left the room, he turned to Erin and said something extraordinary, "Erin, we'll beat the Lions, and then we'll beat everyone else. I promise you that we're going to win the Grey Cup, we're going to win it all."

We made nothing of it at the time. Who doesn't want to win the Grey Cup? In the small eight-team league, the Riders had as good a chance as any other team, but they still had a long way to go to fulfill that promise. We shook hands with Yo and Kerry and wished them good luck. Erin and I said our goodbyes and jokingly said that the next time we see them they better be wheeling the Grey Cup through the hospital hallways.

Erin's Aunt Cindy was the first of our immediate relatives to get her genetics results back. Thankfully, Cindy tested negative for the CDH1 mutation. Erin was very happy to hear it.

★ ★ ★

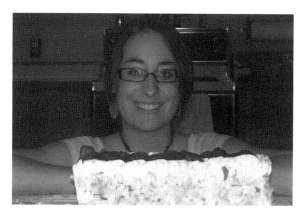

Age 20 –Erin's last birthday

It was now August. Erin's birthday was right around the corner, but she remained very ill and would be spending her 21st birthday in the hospital. Her friends and I agreed to make arrangements to throw Erin a small party in the hospital. I couldn't think of a gift I could give Erin. The only gift I wanted to give her was the only one I couldn't afford, to trade places, to give her, her life back. Even as a hypothetical, I knew Erin probably wouldn't accept that gift, for one simple reason, she loved me too much. I would have gladly taken her place, but in all likelihood, she wouldn't have let me.

I finally came up with an idea. I went to a Riders store in a local mall and asked them whether I could get a jersey personalized with Erin's nickname "Chief" and the number seven on the back, and that I needed it as soon as possible. I told them that it wasn't just Erin's birthday in a few days, but that there was a good possibility she might not live to celebrate it. The lady at the counter called directly to the main office at Mosaic Stadium and ordered the jersey that minute. In a few short hours, it was ready to be picked up. I will always remember those people who made a difference for us.

Officially, "Chief " didn't turn twenty-one until August 7th, but we decided to celebrate Erin's birthday a few days early so that many of Erin's closest friends could make it. As it was a special occasion, I asked the nurses if we could make use of the Solarium in Palliative Care, just around the corner from our room in Ward 3B. The Solarium, as its name suggests, was decorated with all kinds of paintings and plants, sporting comfy modern furniture and a massive glass roof.

That day the sky was absolutely, radiantly, clear. On days like that, the Solarium seemed like the kind of place that helps you forget you're in a hospital. I gave Erin her personalized Riders jersey. Five of Erin's girlfriends went in together and bought a friendship ring set with an olive green Peridot, Erin's birthstone, alongside the birthstones of each of the five friends. They didn't know it, but it would be the last time they would see her alive. That ring would be the last gift that Erin would ever receive, but it wouldn't be the last gift that Erin would ever give.

* * *

By August 6th, Erin and I had spent roughly forty-five straight nights in the hospital together. The day before her twenty-first year on this earth, surrounded by the love and support of her family and friends, Erin passed away. My daughter, my Chief, left this world to be reunited with her mother. Erin's pain was gone, her battle with cancer was over. A mixture of sadness and tranquility washed over us as Erin's great Uncle Ed read various passages from the Bible. I remember Psalm 91 the most:

Surely he shall deliver thee from the snare of the fowler, and from the noisome pestilence.

He shall cover thee with his feathers, and under his wings shalt thou trust; his truth shall be thy shield and buckler.

Thou shalt not be afraid of the terror by night, nor for the arrow that flieth by day.

Nor for the pestilence that walketh in darkness; nor for the destruction that wasteth at noonday. There shall no evil befall thee neither shall any plague come nigh thy dwelling.

A daughter, a step-daughter, a big sister, a soulmate, a grand-daughter, a niece, a cousin, a best friend, a co-worker – Erin was an inspiration to everyone she met. She had a way of sharing her life with everyone, and now Erin had one gift that everyone hoped might some day save another person's life. The CDH1 mutation could now be identified in other relatives. Thanks to Erin, a test had been located that could save many lives. We had been given a gift of knowledge and an opportunity to do something about it. Erin Ashley Lawrence will be forever missed, and never forgotten.

That afternoon, Jared and I walked home from the hospital. The summer had been very hot. The air was thick, the fields dry, our souls swept empty to be filled again only with more dust. But, the afternoon Erin passed away, the heat broke, the skies opened, and it began to pour. The whole thing felt biblical, and not a little surreal, and I thought it would be nice if it were really a sign from Erin that she was free from this world, free of the pain she so long endured, that the newest angel was delivering a well-needed shower, granting us poor survivors a taste of her own reprieve.

It was raining so hard the sewer drains couldn't take all of the run-off. Water began flooding the streets. Jared and I didn't really say much to one another. We just walked and walked through the grey curtain and the blank noise of rain hitting everything. A person can only get so wet and then it doesn't matter. So we walked and walked and walked until we got home. Even then, there was no sound between us but the rain.

"Just when the caterpillar thought life was over,
it became a butterfly."
—English Proverb

CODA: Letters for Erin

The following two letters were written by Erin to her Aunt Charlotte.

Wednesday, February 7, 2007
Hi Aunty Charlotte,

Thank you so very much for all your prayers, they are the most important because it's those prayers that are going to heal me, God has my back and the angels are there to make me strong, i know i will be ok after all of this, it's just something i have to battle first, but in the end i know i will go on to do everything and more that i ever wanted to. Thanks again for your thoughts and prayers, and just so u know chemo went well today, so far so good, not too sick yet, i hope i continue to take it weekly, but i also hope its kicks the crap out of this cancer, so whatever happens will happen and if im sick it will all be for the better in the end. I love you always! God Bless!

Love always, *Erin*

Monday, February 12, 2007
Thank you so much Aunty Charlotte!

I was just thinking about u today actually, i was thinking that i hope you're still praying for me, cuz i feel pretty crappy and i just keep thinking that it's all gonna be worth it in the end cuz i know it'll be ok soon! Thanks so much for ur prayers, and by the way i was watching old home movies and i have to say everyone looks pretty funny in the early nineties! but lisa, Nicole, Jared and i always looked cute!

Love you lots, *Erin*

* * *

The following letter was written by Erin's godfather, Terry.

Erin was with our family the day her mother passed. Something happened that will always stay with me. Erin and [her cousin] Lisa were playing and laughing. I cannot remember exactly what they were doing, but they were having fun. All of a sudden Erin let out a cry and began to sob. Shortly after that our telephone rang. We received the news that RoseMarie had passed. At that moment, Charlotte and I looked at each other and realized RoseMarie came to Erin to say goodbye.

Erin always had a smile when I saw her. I had the privilege of coaching her softball team at a very young age. She approached the game with enthusiasm and a smile. She was one of the most polite young people that I have ever encountered. She always asked me about myself when I would go through her till at the grocery store. That is something you don't always see in young people. When I saw Erin near the end, it amazed me how much she was like her mother in dealing with her situation. It brought back a flood of memories. They both dealt with their situation with unbelievable courage and grace always thinking of others and asking about our lives while theirs were in such turmoil.

I wish I would have spent more time with you Erin.
Love, Terry

* * *

Shealynn Prystupa is the little sister of one of Erin's girlfriends, Lindsay. Shaelynn wrote this distinctive speech for her Grade 8 class after Erin passed away.

Why Me, Why Not...?

Good morning/afternoon honourable judges, guests, teachers, and fellow students. Why me, why not...? Today I am going to acknowledge a special friend that I have known my whole life. My special friend was loved by everyone and anyone who knew her was touched by her compassionate, loving personality. Although my special friend is not here to tell her story, if she was this is what I believe she would say.

I miss her so much. My mom sadly passed away on January 6, 1991 from stomach cancer. I was only five years old and my brother was only two years old. It broke her heart to have to leave my dad, my brother, and I. She was a good mom and she was always there for my brother and I. We were her world. As I grew up I was always told how much I looked like her. Even though her presence was not with me while I was growing up she was still always in my heart. When I was a teenager, I wrote poems for and about my mom. One of these poems is:

"A Deadly Disease"

A mother with a deadly disease has no hope any longer.
She will be gone soon leaving her family and kids.
Why can't there be more time?
To see them grow up and to be with them.
She will be gone soon.
Watching from above, keeping them safe
with her unconditional love.

In some ways, writing the poems made me feel closer to my mom.

After of years of accepting her loss I find myself at the age of twenty years old and diagnosed with cancer. It was a hard seven months. I was diagnosed with cancer on January 6th, 2007. The type of cancer I had is rare and fast growing. My cancer affected my esophagus and stomach. Then it spread to my bones, spine, and brain. A number of different treatments were tried, including radiation and chemotherapy but those just did not seem to work. Genetic testing was done on my mom's side of the family in hopes that if anyone else got it, it could be treated more successfully in earlier stages than mine was. My grandma and brother both tested positive to being carriers of the gene that has caused my stomach cancer. Cancer is a horrible disease and I wish that nobody would have to suffer through it. So I ask myself? Why me? I'm young; I have my whole life ahead of me, but then why not me. There are many other good people out there who are very ill who probably feel the same way as I do. I guess we must wait to see what God's purpose is. Through my strong belief in God I remained optimistic.

My friends and I have a bond that will last forever in life and death. Many of them have been my friends since early childhood. When I was in the hospital, my friends were always with me and they also made custom orange bracelets that showed their love for me. Even though my cancer was advanced, my friends and I would still try to have fun. On July 1st, we had a big bash out at my beach. After I passed away my friends, loved ones, and the elementary school I went to raised money for a memorial bench and trees to be put in Westhill Park. I could not live without my friends.

I cannot believe the Saskatchewan Roughriders did this for me. Someone advised their office of my situation and then did many things for me. One of the games against the Edmonton Eskimos, the Riders dedicated the game to me. They ended up winning the game and presented me with the game ball and other memorabilia. The quarterback then dedicated his season to me and wore the same orange bracelet that all my friends and family wear. He never took it off for the entire season. It was such an honour for the team to do this for me.

It all happened on August 6, 2007. I passed away with all of my friends and family around me. I was sent up to heaven to be reunited with my mother. My funeral was on August 11, 2007, at 2:00 p.m. There were many people there that came along with many tears. At my graveside service, my spirit found a connection with nature. A frog decided to join me in my body's resting place, it reassured me even after death my body will not be alone. The frog hopping in before my body had descended proved significant for I will not be going in alone. At about the same time the sun came pouring out from behind some huge clouds. It broke my heart to see my loved ones have to say goodbye to me.

Why did they have to go through this? My dad and brother both have to go through the loss of a wife, a mom, a daughter, and a sister. My brother has had to go through some medical treatments to prevent getting the same cancer as our mom and I. He has good days and bad days but by far he is doing well. For my dad, stepmom, and brother they take it one day at a time. Some days are harder than others to get through. They have a lot of joyous memories of the wonderful times we shared. Together they will be strong.

My special friend does not represent just myself, but all of us. We need to understand that things can be so much worse. Although many people suffered the loss of my special friend we now have gained the comfort of an angel watching over us. She taught us valuable lessons of the importance of life and cherishing what you have. My special friend opened up my eyes for the significance of life, now I challenge you to find your own inspiration. By Shealynn N. D. Prystupa

* * *

The following emails were sent from the author to the local newspaper, The Leader-Post. *A transcription of the story that eventually made its way into that paper follows .*

From: Luke Lawrence
To: Vanstone, Rob (The Leader-Post)
Sent: Friday, October 05, 2007 3:47 PM
Subject: Thank You Kerry Joseph

Kerry Joseph is more than a quarterback for the Saskatchewan Roughriders. He is a leader and inspiration to this community and the people around him. Let me explain what I mean.

Mr. Joseph took it upon himself to personally make good on his promise to my daughter, Erin Lawrence, who passed away of stomach cancer on Aug. 6th. Mr. Joseph visited Erin in the hospital the day before and the day after the Roughriders defeated the Edmonton Eskimos 54-14 on July 28th, and he gave her a game ball after the victory. Erin's wish was enough to inspire Kerry Joseph and change his life forever. They pounded the Eskimos and put forth a winning streak that is leading this province into playoff frenzy. Only a few people really know what motivates this amazing, talented young man. Kerry Joseph wears a bright orange wristband as a tribute to Erin's memory. Only family and friends wear this band.

Kerry Joseph is the most personable man we have ever met. He wears his heart on his sleeve.

He is much more to us than the Saskatchewan Roughriders' quarterback. Our family has great respect for him. On behalf of the Lawrence family, we cannot thank Kerry Joseph enough. He is sincere and a great leader. Although they met twice in the hospital, Erin and Kerry have a lot in common. It is never about them, but what they can do for you. I want to publicly thank Kerry Joseph for what he has done for Erin and wearing her wristband demonstrates how blessed we are. Bring home the Grey Cup.

God bless, *Luke Lawrence*

From: Luke Lawrence
To: Vanstone, Rob (The Leader-Post)
Sent: Thursday, October 04, 2007 9:24 AM
Subject: Article re Erin Lawrence

I rec'd a phone call this a.m. from a friend in Saskatoon re: an article in the Saskatoon Star Phoenix. I scrambled to the mailbox and discovered that the front page of the sports section of the Leader Post read, "Lawrence Touched Joseph's Heart". After reading the article, we literally broke down. I presented Kerry Joseph and Yo Murphy with keepsakes in honour of Erin's memory at a Riders practice. Kerry greeted me with open arms with tears in his eyes. He apologized for not being able to attend Erin's funeral, as the team was en route back from Toronto.

Kerry Joseph is the most personable man we have ever met. He wears his heart on his sleeve. He is much more to us than the Saskatchewan Roughrider's quarterback. Our family has great respect for this talented young man. Erin's wish was for the "Riders to pound the Eskimos" and beat the Lions. The Roughriders fulfilled her wish. On behalf of the Lawrence family, we cannot thank Kerry Joseph enough. He is sincere and a great leader. Although they met twice in the hospital, Erin and Kerry have a lot in common. It is never about them, but what they can do for you. He has been an inspiration to all of us. We are just beginning to find out how much Erin has changed a lot of lives since her passing. Erin, too wore her heart on her sleeve. *Now Kerry Joseph wears Erin's armband on his sleeve.* We thank you for your article and consider it a great honour in Erin's memory.

God Bless
Thank You
Luke Lawrence

Lawrence touched Joseph's heart

Erin's Gift

The Leader-Post (Regina)
Thu Oct 4 2007
Page: C1 / FRONT
Section: Sports
Byline: Rob Vanstone
Source: The Leader-Post

Kerry Joseph is accustomed to being a recipient of fan adoration. However, the roles can occasionally be reversed.

The Saskatchewan Roughriders quarterback quickly became an admirer of Erin Lawrence -- a terminally ill cancer patient whose final days were enhanced by Joseph.

Lawrence died Aug. 6, one day before her 21st birthday, from the same form of stomach cancer that claimed her mother at age 29.

The courageous Lawrence left such an impression on Joseph that he wears an "I Love Erin" wristband during games.

"She's someone I was really blessed to meet," Joseph said Wednesday after he was named the CFL's offensive player-of-the-week for the third time this season. "It was just an opportunity to go and meet a big fan of ours who was fighting for her life.

"It just touched my heart to see her spirit. People in her situation, knowing there's no cure, could really be down in the dumps but she was a real high-spirited person. All she wanted us to do was go out and win as a team and go on and win the Grey Cup. Just meeting her and seeing her attitude really touched my life.

"You go through so much in life that sometimes you complain about the little things and you don't realize how blessed we are. Just to meet her family and see the support that they give to us, it was just an honour."

Joseph, who turns 34 today, was introduced to Lawrence the day after one of her friends contacted the Roughriders. The community-minded quarterback visited her at Pasqua Hospital on July 27 -- one day before Saskatchewan defeated the Edmonton Eskimos 54-14 on Taylor Field.

The following day, Joseph returned to the hospital with teammate Yo Murphy and presented Lawrence with a game ball and some autographed Roughriders paraphernalia. In turn, Joseph was given the wristband.

Lawrence died nine days later. Joseph responded by writing a letter to the family, telling Lawrence's loved ones about the lasting imprint she left in such a short time.

"Erin fought her cancer from the beginning to the end," Lindsay Prystupa, one of Lawrence's best friends, said via e-mail from Cranbrook, B.C. "She never let her cancer get in the way.

"She went camping on the May long weekend, had season tickets for the Riders, enrolled in her classes for the U of R in the fall, and she had a trip planned to Edmonton for the Keith Urban concert.

"She never complained about the pain, and would even crack a joke. Even as her pain progressed, she was more concerned about others than her own cancer. Even if we had a stomach ache or a simple headache, Erin would feel worse for us than herself."

Prystupa and another one of Lawrence's friends, Megan Mohr, met Joseph when the Roughriders visited Calgary for a Sept. 15 game against the Stampeders. Prystupa and Mohr were so grateful to discover that Joseph was still wearing and cherishing the "I Love Erin" wristband.

Jill Wenzel, another one of Lawrence's friends, met Joseph while he was signing autographs last week at the Woman's World trade show. When Wenzel mentioned Lawrence's name, Joseph responded: "She changed my life."

"It kind of reminded me of when I lost my dad -- just seeing her in the hospital and seeing that smile on her face, knowing that everything was going to be all right," said the devout Joseph, whose father died of congestive heart failure. "She was a Christian girl, so she knew she was at peace with her situation. She had lost her mom to the same illness.

"It was a humbling experience and it's something that I hold dear to me. It's something they didn't ask for, but it's part of life. You just want to pray for them and keep them in your spirit."

The same attitude is maintained by Lawrence's circle of friends -- the closest of which were Prystupa, Mohr, Nicole Sarauer, Ali Pulvermacher and Tricia Fluter.

"Erin is an inspiration to us all, for we are very grateful for having been so lucky to be friends with her," Prystupa concluded.

"Erin is now the wings on our backs and will forever be with us."

★ ★ ★

To Erin

Erin left this world to be in a better place. Erin's mother was her mentor in Life. Losing her mom when she was a little girl inspired Erin to see life in a *special* way. It molded her into a loving caring person we all admired. Erin loved and treated everyone equally. She loved people and always put the people in her life first. "It's not meant for us to understand in this life-time." *Love Kerry Joseph*

★ ★ ★

My dearest Erin,

Our life is not the same without you in our lives and a lot has happened since you left us! I'm sure you know all about it. They say things happen for a reason. Only you have an answer for that. I'm sure you are in heaven with your mother; I know she is proud of the things you have done in the short time we shared our lives together. Please say hello to your mom and grandpa for me. I know that you know how long our journey will be before we meet again. I ask that God grant me your gift. I hope to use this gift to help other people and be an example of what you have taught me. I thank you for helping me write my book and giving me the strength to finish it. Words cannot express my loss; a part of me has died, and a part of me will always be with you. Erin, you were our lamb. You made the ultimate sacrifice and gave the ultimate gift to your family. *Thank you for saving your brother's life.* GOD BLESS.

All my love, Dad

★ ★ ★

The following, mostly anonymous, testimonials were written by Erin's family and friends at her funeral.

To Erin & Brett – a perfect love! If only I could have said happy 6th anniversary today!! I miss so much the friendship and love the two of you shared.
Miss you more than anything muffin, I hate having to bring a new year in without you, but I know you're always with me. Keep meeting me in my dreams. Love you forever pumpkin. (L)

• Wish you were here…

• I talked to Kerry Joseph right after the Grey Cup was over. He had his I ♥ ERIN bracelet on and when he saw mine he came over and said "It's all because of Erin. If it wasn't for her beside me the entire game we wouldn't have won.

She's the reason we played the way we did, the entire team wanted to win it for her and we did."

- Riders win because of you hun, I know you had everything to do with it.

- Love you girl, forever!

- There's not much more I can write here that hasn't been said about Erin already. She was a pleasure to know and truly a great person. Even while she was going through treatment you would never know; other than her physical changes she was the same upbeat person all the time. I knew her since she was just a baby when her and my sis were running around in their diapers. Even now when I'm at my parents' I sometimes still expect to see her out the back window at her house. You were like a little sister to me and you will always be missed and remembered.

- Erin you are never far from my thoughts. You were my daughter, a perfect friend and everything a mother could want for her son. I miss your bright and beautiful smile that graced our house daily. I miss our talks and will treasure all the moments that I was blessed to share with you. You made my life so complete. I can't seem to find a way out of sadness. The house is empty and there are constant reminders (which I am so grateful for). You were so precious and genuine – there will never be another you! Thank you for leaving me in such good hands. I can understand why you picked your best friends. They, like you, are genuine, kind and loving and make me feel that I still have a living part of you with me. I love you sweet girl and miss you so much!

- A charismatic person is defined as possessing an extraordinary ability to attract; a magnetic personality. Only a few people in the world are known to be like this, including Princess Diana and Ghandi. Erin is the only one I personally knew who had this special characteristic. Anyone who ever met Erin was just drawn to her, it is unexplainable. She was an angel living among us on Earth. There is not much I can say of Erin that has not been said already, but I think of her every day and miss her more and more. I know she cannot be here with me on Earth anymore but I still see her in my dreams and all around me. She was an amazing, beautiful girl inside and out and will be in my heart forever. I miss you Erin.

- Erin... I knew her barely, but I heard a lot of positive things from friends and many others that know her. I believe that when someone goes to heaven they are always watching you, and that is truly how I feel about Erin. She was a gorgeous girl. I only met her twice in my life, and in those two times I thought she was the nicest person EVER! Erin, you were loved by so many people. See you soon.

- I only knew Erin from school and classes she was in with me, she was the most selfless, kindest person I have ever met. Erin was so happy and positive; I believe she is an example of how every one of us should try to live our lives; to treat everyone the same with respect and be positive no matter what we're going through. R.I.P Erin

- I will never forget Erin. I spent a lot of time as a youngster with her. We would help her dad build awesome haunted houses in the garage and build crafts at my house around Christmas and many other holidays. To this day she has the M&M wreath we made at Christmas one year... I wish I would not have lost touch with her, but the time I did was unforgettable. Erin has such a kind heart, always putting others ahead of her. She truly is the most beautiful person inside and out I have ever met and I'm sure will ever meet.

- I feel so blessed to have known Erin! I've never known anyone so strong, compassionate and truly pure of heart, as Erin! She really is an angel!!

- There won't ever be a day that I won't think of her. She had a huge impact on me and many others. I find myself constantly contemplating my actions, asking myself what

Erin would do. We can all learn tremendously from her. I love you forever Erin!

- Erin, wow, where do I begin, she such a strong, passionate and caring person, words can't describe the kind of person Erin is. She is an Angel!! Even at her hardest of times she was more concerned for everyone else. She is greatly missed and loved so much by everyone she knew. Erin has touched so many lives with her uplifting spirits and strong outlook in life. Having the opportunity of Erin being my first best friend is priceless, I couldn't have asked for a better person! She is great! Erin you will never be forgotten for all the great things you did throughout your life .

- Erin was an amazing person. She was so strong and brave, and she never let anything slow her down. She is always on my mind, and I think about her every day. She has impacted everyone who knew her and will never be forgotten.

- It's quite obvious Erin was my 2nd older sister... but in May I got in a stupid bar fight and ended up with a broken nose, two black eyes. Erin came over the next day and was so concerned about how I was that I said, "Me? How are you?" I realize now it was rude of me to be like that but in the long run... that's just how Erin was. No matter the circumstances she put everyone else before herself... and that's how she'll always be remembered.

- Erin has touched the lives of so many. She was with me before I was born, and when I was she would babysit me. She always had a positive attitude and was willing to help others in need of help. Even when she was in pain she cared for others around her. We all love her and will be in my heart forever and ever.

- Erin has been a huge part of my life. She is truly an inspiration and always will be. Erin had every quality you could ever ask for in a friend. I am missing her every minute of the day, there is not a day goes by that she is not on my mind. Erin had the heart, smile, eyes, and gentle loving touch of an angel. Erin will always be in my heart.

- Erin was the greatest person I ever met, one of the most compassionate and one of the bravest. Not a second of any day goes by where I'm not thinking about her. She will never be forgotten and the only thing we can do is to live our lives in a way that would make her proud, and to fill it with as much happiness as possible.

- Erin, you will forever be in my thoughts. I see you in so many places; usually guarding over my daughters. This world is a much better place because you were here. I can only hope to make a difference in my time here as well. We have learned so much from you in such a short time. Thanks for allowing me to be a part of your life.

- Erin you are a rare and precious gift to all your family and friends. You have always had the ability to put others first and tune in to just what they need. You helped a lot of people here on earth and you continue to help from above. I have had to draw on your strength many times.

- You are a true Christian and the world would be a wonderful place if we could follow in your footsteps. I miss you and your mom more than words can ever say; you lost your mom at such a young age, but you always had a special bond with her. You are in my thoughts every day, sometimes with laughter and sometimes with tears. I feel both of your presence and know you are still with us, just in a different way. I would love to give you one of those Auntie Mel hugs!! I think it's your mom's turn to have the precious gift – she waited a long time. Knowing you and your mom are together now gets me through the tough times. Life's accomplishments aren't measured by the length of time we are here on Earth.

- I truly believe I have a guardian angel, when things are going bad something always reminds me of Erin that makes me feel better. I learned a lot from Erin, even though she was only here a short time; she lived life to the fullest and didn't dwell on the small things. No matter what, she always put others before herself and that made her an extraordinary girl. She was a great person and is missed by many people but I know she is looking down on everyone with that huge smile of hers. I will never forget you Erin you're my inspiration and I hope I can be half the person you were. Love, your cousin, Mike

- Erin was the greatest person I ever met, one of the most compassionate and one of the bravest. Not a second of any day goes by where I'm not thinking about her. She will never be forgotten and the only thing we can do is to live our lives in a way that would make her proud, and to fill it with as much happiness as possible. - J

- I only had the chance to meet Erin a few times, but those moments have stayed with me. She was truly inspirational. She was a tremendous spirit, who had such compassion and care for everyone around her. Her spirit has clearly brought so much joy to everyone who shared in her life and will continue to, I am sure.

- It's hard to put into words the impact this young lady had on others. Her spirit lives on and I truly believe that she was put on this earth by God to help us by showing us how precious life is, how to be a good person, how to feel the pain of losing a loved one and how to live with that and have her spirit guide us towards positives by not becoming hateful or bitter. Erin would not have tolerated that, she wants us to grow from her death, carry on, learn, teach others by searching our own soul. God gives you only what you can handle, he has a plan for everyone. Our life is a journey and everything that happens has meaning. Be patient... you will understand one day... why we hurt so much. Erin's life and death has certainly made me personally search deep within and help me to walk a path of richer fulfillment. It hurts, I want to talk to her, I want to see her. I have not yet found the understanding of her death, but I will be patient Erin as I continue to search with your help. I miss you every day.

- Erin was not only my cousin but she was my best friend. She knew everything about me and helped me through a lot of hard times. Any time I needed somebody to talk to she was there for me. She always knew what to say to make me feel better. In my mind, Erin was as close to perfect as possible, she was an angel and no one will ever be able to replace her. Everybody mattered to Erin – Ashley

Part Three:
TOWARDS THE NEW NORMAL

Chapter Seventeen

THE FUNERAL SERVICE

We decided that like RoseMarie's service, Erin's prayer service would be held in Regina, on August 9, 2007 and her funeral service in Rocanville on August 11th. Erin's friends celebrated her life by creating a collage of photographs that they put to music, a time capsule of memories. Erin loved country music. I thought it would be appropriate to choose a song that she loved and that would in some small way capture something of her life. I decided on "The Dance" by Garth Brooks, a beauty of a song about memory, loss, perfect moments, unpredictability, how things could be otherwise, how we never see what's coming. *"Yes, my life is better left to chance / I could have missed the pain but I'd have had to miss the dance."* The greatest happiness is inextricably mingled with the pain of its unbearable fragility, its inevitable loss. There's no holding onto it and there's no way to know how long it will last.

Erin's prayer service was held in the church that she grew up attending. It was a powerful experience to see over five hundred people in attendance. I was surprised to see that Dr. Malik and some of the nurses from the hospital were there; it didn't seem to be standard procedure for a surgeon to attend their patient's funeral. But Dr. Malik seemed as emotional as I was and when I approached him, he squeezed me so hard he almost lifted my feet off the floor. It was a Thursday and I was wondering why he wasn't in surgery. I loved his answer: *"Today, everything else will just have to wait."*

Just as with RoseMarie, I asked the pallbearers to carry Erin's casket high above their shoulders. Erin's dance was cut short in life, she was too much like her mother: they were dealt the same hand. On August 11th we laid Erin to rest beside RoseMarie at Webster's Cemetery in Rocanville. To show my appreciation to all those people who made the two-hour journey, I ordered two hundred orange I ♥ ERIN wrist bands and asked two of Erin's best friends to distribute them to people as they entered the church. One of Erin's friends, Vinny had recently graduated the academy to become an officer for the Royal Canadian Mounted Police (RCMP), so I asked if he would be a pallbearer and honour us by wearing his special red "serge," or ceremonial uniform. The father of one of Erin's other friends, a retired RCMP officer, likewise honoured the occasion by wearing his serge. Another of Erin's friends in the Military Reserves wore his army uniform. At Erin's graveside, Vinny approached us and said that he and a few others had prepared something special. He asked permission to go ahead with it, and naturally, I said yes. In Erin's honour, Vinny and two others performed an Honour Guard salute.

Sometimes we can't find the words to express the things we are trying to say. Life is puzzling, we spend a lifetime assembling the pieces. I think Erin had some special piece that everyone needed, albeit in different ways. If things happen for a reason, then I guess Erin was that reason – she touched our lives forever. She had a gift and shared her love with all she met. She had a special compassion that made her feel for others in a way that most of us only feel for ourselves.

She approached life with a smile and always left you with a good impression. She had a way of making sense of the most complex situations. Many of the medical professionals who had met Erin in her battle against the disease told me they would remember her always. I also know that Mr. Joseph was inspired the day he met Erin, and that he always will be. Erin only met with Joseph twice, but each time they passed a gift to one another. The first time it seemed as though Erin had given Mr. Joseph a clearer understanding of how precious life is.

The second time they met, Mr. Joseph brought the Saskatchewan Roughriders to Erin. He and Yo Murphy gave her the ball from their last game against the Eskimos. Erin had said that they were an inspiration for her. Wide-eyed, Mr. Murphy replied, "No, Erin, you're an inspiration for us." The Roughriders were in Toronto the week of Erin's funeral to prepare for their next game. We received a message to pick up a letter from the Rider office from Kerry Joseph, who would be unable to attend Erin's service.

After Erin's funeral, Jared and I stayed in Rocanville and visited his grandparents and met with a dizzying array of friends, uncles, aunts, and cousins. After about a week, Jared and I decided we needed to get away. We drove six hours from Regina to Amisk Lake, a large freshwater lake near the Manitoba border, for a three-day fishing trip. Even though we had three days of nonstop rain, we enjoyed it.

The fish were biting and between the two of us we caught our limit of Northern Pike and were a few shy of our limit in Walleye. Jared's test results had been available for over a month, but we had postponed heading to Saskatoon to meet with the geneticists because of Erin's condition. Between bites, Jared and I discussed his options. He told me that if he carried the gene, he had already had made a decision as to what we would do next, but he didn't say what that decision would be. The immediate next step would be to go to Saskatoon and meet with Katherine.

On August 20th, Erin's grandmother received her test results. It was as we expected: positive. The results confirmed that Erin's grandma was a carrier of the disease from her parents and their ancestors. It had been suspected that her grandfather had also passed away from stomach cancer.

Chapter Eighteen

TEENAGE WRISTBANDS

"Just meeting her and seeing her attitude really touched my life."
—Kerry Joseph

I wanted to give Mr. Joseph and Yo Murphy a keepsake from Erin's service, so one afternoon I went to watch the Riders practice at Mosaic Stadium. I told the Riders' media person who I was and asked if I could speak with Kerry after practice. He told me he would give Kerry the message right away.

I hung around for about an hour watching the team practice from the stands. While I was there, I struck up a conversation with a man who introduced himself as Glen Reid, a sports anchor with CBC television who was there to interview some of the players after practice. I wondered why an anchor would be doing interviews, and Reid began to explain how cutbacks had forced some of the anchors to do their own reporting. He asked me if I usually came to a lot of practices. I said that I didn't.

I told Mr. Reid a little about Erin's passing and her short but special friendship with Joseph. I was only there that day to give Joseph and Murphy Erin's obituary and a commemorative wristband. After practice was over, the media all gathered to one side of the field, waiting to interview some of the players. Kerry Joseph and Yo Murphy emerged from the practice field, they spotted me standing behind a small crowd of jostling reporters and cameramen. They dropped their equipment and walked straight through the media scrum to greet me. As Joseph embraced me with a great big hug, I noticed Mr. Reid signal his cameraman to start rolling.

I knew that I had come for the right reasons. I knew that Erin would have wanted me to do this.

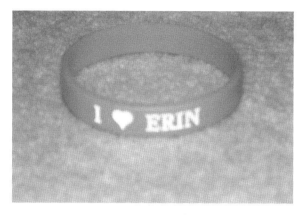

I ♥ ERIN wristband

I handed Joseph and Murphy each an envelope that contained a copy of Erin's obituary and an I ♥ ERIN wristband to remember her by. I thanked them both for taking the time to talk with me, for coming into Erin's life at such a difficult time and making her last few weeks so memorable. Joseph had tears in his eyes while we spoke. Before we said our goodbyes, he reiterated his promise to Erin, "We're going to win the Grey Cup, I'm going to do it for her."

Mr. Reid captured the moment and later sent me a copy of the tape. Although the footage never aired, our story was expanding beyond our family and friends. I hope Erin's story will raise awareness about HDGC on a wider scale.

As the final week of August approached, Jan, Jared, Jared's girlfriend Kimberly, and I all drove to Saskatoon to discuss the results of Jared's genetic test. We knew from previous consultations that a person had a 50/50 chance of inheriting the bad copy from a carrier parent and developing HDGC, and that once inherited, a male had a sixty-seven per cent lifetime chance of developing diffuse gastric cancer. In the car, I noticed Jared flipping a coin: *heads I win, tails you lose.*

The four of us made our way to the clinic and waited in a small room furnished with a couch and two chairs for what seemed like a very long time. The longer we waited, the more nervous we became. Finally, Katherine and Dr. Lemire walked into the room. We felt like we were the accused, waiting for jurors to announce our verdict. We could see it in her eyes before she even spoke: *guilty.* Jared had tested positive for the mutation. Both Katherine and Dr. Lemire came out strongly in favour of a prophylactic gastrectomy.

We asked questions regarding Jared's age and the surgery, but no answers were immediately forthcoming. There was no history of a person Jared's age having this surgery. We were also told that Erin was reported to have been the youngest person in North America in 2007 to have passed away from the disease. We were wandering into uncharted territory, and we were carrying a map without coordinates. On September 5th, another relative received their genetic test results: Aunt Melodie tested negative.

The following week we contacted Dr. Malik's office and told him that Jared had decided to go ahead with the surgery. Royal University Hospital in Saskatoon was going to forward a letter to him confirming that Jared had inherited the CDH1 mutation. Jan and I arranged to meet with Dr. Malik in confidence, away from the tense atmosphere of his office at the hospital. He said he had been hoping for better news, but would offer us his services or, if we preferred another opinion, he had no problem referring Jared to another doctor. Jared's opinion, however, was that if Dr. Malik was good enough for Erin, he would be good enough for him. We went ahead and booked Jared's surgery for September 19th.

I initially wanted to get another opinion for Jared just as we did for Erin, but I knew from what we had already gone through that Jared had the opportunity to have surgery before the CDH1 mutation could develop into HDGC, an opportunity Erin herself never had. Erin's death wasn't to be in vain. She had given her brother Jared a *gift* and a chance to beat this cancer!

Chapter Nineteen
THE CONFERENCE CALL

September 13th – Katherine had arranged a conference call between Dr. Huntsman, Dr. Lynch and us. They advised Jared to postpone the surgery until he reached the age of twenty. They felt that he was still growing and this could complicate matters since, after the removal of the stomach, Jared would no longer be able to absorb enough Vitamin B12 to continue to grow at all. One of the doctors asked Jared how tall he was and Jared's only response was that he would rather be "short and alive than tall and dead."

The doctors had no knowledge of anyone Jared's age ever having a pro-phylactic gastrectomy. At eighteen years of age, Jared was unofficially (at least until medical journals confirmed it) the youngest person to ever have this type of surgery. Given the doctors' overall caution, Jan and I decided it might be best to try and get a hold of Dr. Bathe for another opinion. When we contacted his office, we were told he was currently on sabbatical. This would make it impossible for us to get a hold of him on the phone, so we decided to send him an e-mail.

A few days later, another one of Erin's relatives, an uncle, received the results of his genetic test, which also came back negative. This was the fourth set of results to come back. In case you're keeping score: Erin's grandma had tested positive, while two aunts and an uncle had tested negative. We were still waiting on one uncle, two great uncles and one great aunt.

Because I had spent almost as much time in the hospital in the past year as the people who worked there, I had noticed a couple of things that I thought could be improved to make patient care a bit easier for everyone involved. The first thing I noticed was that the waiting room at the Allan Blair Cancer Centre had nothing to offer patients and others to pass the time except outdated magazines that had been donated from mysterious sources (it was more interesting to daydream about the people whose names often still adorned the address labels on the back of the magazines themselves – who was "Mrs. X" and what was she looking for in a 1998 *Good Housekeeping* prominently featuring Meryl Streep? Who is "Mr. Y" and what did he make of a 1999 *Sports Illustrated* that proclaimed the New York Mets infield from that season the 'best ever'). It was either the magazines or chewing your fingernails to the bone, as I did. The second thing I noticed was that the cancer ward had only one full size fridge located in the galley area for everyone to use. So after Erin passed away, I spent the remaining portions of Erin's fundraising and purchased eight compact fridges for Ward 3B and a 32-inch plasma TV for the Allan Blair's waiting room, each bearing a small golden plaque inscribed with the words "In Memory of Erin Lawrence."

On September 18th, we received a phone call from Dr. Bathe. As we began our conversation concerning the possibility of Jared having his stomach removed at such a young age, our second line began ringing. Asking Dr. Bathe to hold, I clicked over and heard the familiar voice of Dr. Malik. Sounding as though he was fighting to keep his emotions in check, Dr. Malik said he had decided he would not perform Jared's surgery. He felt he had become personally involved and was too close to the situation. I explained to Dr. Malik that Dr. Bathe was currently on the other line and asked if he would like to speak with him. I put Dr. Malik on hold and asked Dr. Bathe if he would agree to a conference call with Dr. Malik. There was a short pause before Dr. Bathe, in a somewhat baffled tone said, "What... right now?"

I told him that Dr. Malik was, indeed, on the other line that very moment. Dr. Bathe – still sounding a bit puzzled – agreed and I put Dr. Malik through. The doctors began discussing Jared's situation. Dr. Malik explained his reservations about doing the surgery himself and asked if Dr. Bathe would possibly accept his referral. We collectively held our breaths. We knew Dr. Bathe was the next best thing, but we weren't sure what he would say. There was a long pause.

Finally, Dr. Bathe broke through the blank hum of the telephone line. He explained that because he was currently on sabbatical, he would have to contact one of his associates, Dr. Mack, to see if he would agree to perform the surgery while he (Dr. Bathe) would assist. Dr. Bathe assured us that Dr. Mack would get back to us shortly while Dr. Malik agreed to send out a letter of referral the next day. Needless to say, Jan and I were a bit astonished at what had just happened. What were the chances that, while we were on the phone with Dr. Bathe – itself something of a shot in the dark given that he was on sabbatical – Dr. Malik would happen to call at the very same time? It couldn't have worked out better if we had planned it (indeed, if we *had* tried to plan a conference call between these two very busy doctors it likely would never have happened). I had a sense that, for once, fate had actually worked in our favour, that our *"Chief"* was looking over her brother's shoulder that day.

We told Jared what had just happened and he was, understandably, upset. He had been mentally preparing himself to go in for surgery the next day, a surgery that was now postponed until further notice. I told him that, all things considered, we were incredibly lucky things happened the way they did. But Jared was still worried, since no replacement date had been set up. Certainty had given way to uncertainty, yet again. Summer browned into autumn. The doctors kept us informed about possible surgery dates and what kind of recovery time would be expected.

Recovery would have to last a full year, meaning that Jared would not be able to continue at work or with his university studies for at least that long. Jared's girlfriend, Kimberly, her parents, Erin's friend Nikki's mother Donna, and Lyn, all decided to organize a fundraiser to help Jared after his surgery. The owners of a local Boston Pizza in Regina graciously donated their staff and their restaurant for the event, which was a great success. Most everyone who knew Erin and Jared stopped in at some point to show their support. Even Jared's old high school football coach showed up, and brought along the current edition of the football team that Jared had been a part of for four years.

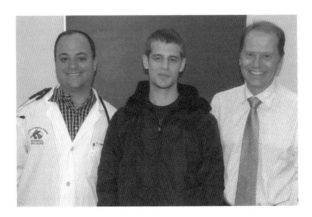

Dr. Mack, Jared, and Dr. Bathe

A little less than two weeks later, Jan, Jared and I flew to Calgary for a consultation with Dr. Bathe and Dr. Mack, who finally set a date for Jared's surgery. Dr. Bathe then explained the risk factors involved in performing a surgery of this kind on someone as young as Jared. Dr. Bathe informed us that a total gastrectomy surgery carried with it an approximatly one per cent mortality rate, Jared responded by saying that having a one per cent chance of dying from the surgery seemed to pale in comparison to the seventy per cent chance he had of developing the disease.

Chapter Twenty

SURGERY IN CALGARY

We decided we would travel to Calgary by car, and arrived two days prior to Jared's surgery. A woman named Karen Humphrey had arranged for us to stay in the Foothills Medical Centre Patient Hostel at the Foothills Medical Centre, which was located on the twelfth and thirteenth floors of the South Tower Building on the main campus, directly across from the Tom Baker Cancer Centre. The day we arrived we went out for supper, giving Jared a last opportunity to really fill his stomach. In a couple of days, all of it would be gone.

One of the risks that Dr. Bathe and Dr. Mack had warned us about was that with the total removal of the stomach, there was a possibility of bile reflux from the upper part of the small intestine into the esophagus.

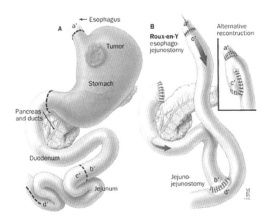

Illustration of Roux-en-Y

To prevent this, the surgeons would be performing the cumbrously named Roux-en-Y esophagojejunostomy. Besides sounding like the name of an alien race on Star Trek or an especially secret martial arts technique, Roux-en-Y esophagojejunostomy describes a method of surgical reconstruction in which the part of the small bowel that is initially cut at the end of the duodenum – the lower end of intestine (jejunum) – is extended straight up to meet the esophagus. The cut end of the duodenum is then reconnected to the small bowel to ensure the regular flow of bile from the duodenum into the lower intestine, rather than back up through the esophagus.

The procedure itself would take four to five hours, followed by a hospital stay of seven to twelve days. To prepare ourselves, Jan and I began roaming through various discussion groups on the Internet, trying to get a more complete picture of what we might expect from life after surgery. We knew Jared would not be allowed to eat or drink, only be able to suck on ice cubes for the first couple of days after the surgery. The "new plumbing" needed time to heal, and any kind of leakage through the jejunum into the esophagus was potentially lethal.

Jared would have to wait three or four days before any solid food would be permitted. The discussion groups uniformly confirmed that the first eight weeks after surgery would be the most difficult. Eating itself would become a painful and uncomfortable experience, and many have to force themselves to eat anything whatsoever. Thirty to sixty minutes after eating, most said they would experience symptoms of nausea, cramps, and diarrhea because of the near instantaneous and unmediated passage of food into the small intestine. Due to rapid spikes and crashes in blood sugar levels, one might likewise experience sweating, increased heart rate, and weakness between 1-1/2 hours to 3 hours after meals. Hunger no longer exists, they said. In its place, there is a perpetual feeling of emptiness, a hole right in the centre of your being. Eventually, it was said, a desire to eat would return, but the emptiness would be permanent.

Most symptoms could be controlled through changes in eating habits. To avoid symptoms it was recommended that Jared eat roughly six to eight small meals a day, and try to avoid eating too much at any given time. Drinking something about one-half hour before or after a meal rather than with a meal was also recommended. The permanent loss of close to twenty per cent of total body weight was typically said to occur within the first six months.

Due to the rapidity of weight loss, some patients develop gallstones that necessitate the removal of the gallbladder. Maintaining proper vitamin levels becomes a serious challenge, and consequently, osteoporosis – a reduction of bone-mineral density – also becomes a concern. Chewable vitamins were said to help, as would occasional iron infusions. Without a stomach, the body wouldn't be able to properly absorb Vitamin B12, so monthly B12 shots were also considered critical.

Consuming enough calories to maintain energy levels can be difficult, so one had to be on the lookout for nutritious, high calorie, low-sugar foods. Just finding something like that was in itself a challenge. It was said that the body seemed to adjust to the absence of the stomach in about one to two years. In short, it sounded like the next two years were going to suck.

At 6:00 a.m. on October 24th, Jared, Jan and I walked into the Emergency Department, registered and then hung around the admitting desk until Jared's name was called. We followed a porter to the surgical ward and were led to what would be Jared's room. A nurse came in and went over Jared's file and then asked if he would consider donating his stomach to the lab. Jared said he didn't care what they did with it. He signed some release papers, changed into a hospital gown and off we went. We followed a porter who took us to a waiting area outside of the Operating Room. They handed Jared a thick blanket and told us that his anesthetist would be in to speak with us shortly.

At 8:00 a.m., the waiting room was packed. Two fully gowned and capped female nurses entered the waiting room from a hallway to our left and asked for Jared. I wondered if they were on Jared's surgical team and they responded in the affirmative. They were in fact specialists in this type of surgery. The anesthetist told us that Jared was in good hands and not to worry. Yeah, right. Don't worry. Not bloody likely. Why worry? My eighteen-year-old son was about to become the youngest person to ever have his stomach removed as a precautionary measure against a deadly form of cancer that he had a 50/50 chance of inheriting, a cancer that had already killed my first wife and my only daughter. Don't worry? You'd have to drug me silly to pull that one off, sister.

The nurses asked Jared to follow them. I watched silently as he walked down a hallway, turned right, and disappeared into the Operating Room. I had tears in my eyes; I was so proud of him, proud of his bravery. He was having the surgery that Erin couldn't have, but that she helped make possible. Jan and I were leaving the OR's reception area when, just outside the doors, we bumped into Dr. Mack, who was speeding towards the Operating Room. He asked us if it was okay if another surgeon from down east who happened to be in Calgary doing a seminar on prophylactic gastrectomies, could observe the procedure. I replied with something flip like "the more the merrier." It certainly couldn't hurt. The more expertise in the Operating Room, I figured the better.

It was another instance of fate breaking our way. What were the odds that this particular doctor was in Calgary *that day*, at the very same time in the same hospital giving a seminar on the very type of surgery Jared was about to have? The way things were going, somebody should have bought a lottery ticket.

We returned to the surgical ward we had visited earlier that morning. They told us a special nurse liaison would be assigned to Jared's surgery. She would serve as a go-between throughout Jared's procedure, letting us know of any updates in real time. It was just after two hours into the surgery when the liaison came in and told us that Jared was doing fine under the anaesthetic. A good first step, but a first step only. I couldn't help but watch the clock and think about how Jared had walked straight into the Operating Room, seemingly without any fear, with a hint of defiance.

Some time later, the liaison nurse returned with an update from Dr. Mack. It was a relief to hear that, three-quarters of the way through the surgery, Jared was doing *"amazingly well."* It still didn't stop me from pacing up and down the hall, wondering anxiously how much longer it would take. Every now and then, when I reached the end of the hallway, I would look out of the window to see Calgary's first snowfall of the year.

It was 12:30 p.m. when Dr. Bathe came in to see us. He was still wearing his green operating scrubs when he told us that Dr. Mack was just closing Jared up and that everything had gone very well. I asked him if they had removed a "normal" stomach and he had a smile on his face, "We think so, yes, but we'll have to wait for pathology to confirm everything."

I was so happy I was in tears. Dr. Bathe told me to go outside and take a long walk, as Jared wouldn't be down from Recovery for another couple of hours. I took his advice and did just that I walked around the hospital and outside the campus in the fresh, new fallen snow. I looked up into the falling snowflakes. They looked like feathers from heaven. I closed my eyes and said, "Thank you."

Jan and I went back to the hostel and waited until Jared returned from Recovery. My first impression was that he looked pretty good for someone who no longer had a stomach. We had requested a private room, but they couldn't tell us if one was available, so for the time being, we were stuck with three other patients.

It was a sight I'd seen too many times already. Jared had tubes sticking out of him and IV lines crisscrossing all over his bed. There was an epidural in his back to block the inevitable and oncoming pain. An epidural is a very small tube placed into the spine by the anesthetist in the Operating Room that is connected to an IV line that is hooked into a pump. It releases a very small but continuous amount of, in Jared's case, hydromorphone.

Jared told us as he made his way into the Operating Room, he spied the tray of surgical instruments to be used and said to the nurses, "You should cover that shit up, you've got more tools here than Home Hardware."

Jan and I traded a smile. Despite having just lost his stomach, it didn't appear as though Jared had lost any of his character. Around 5:00 p.m., Jan and I told Jared we would be leaving and see him tomorrow. I was hoping he could sleep off some of the pain. Jan and I would make our way back to the hostel through the underground parkway connected with the hospital, we felt a twinge of guilt when we fixed ourselves something to eat, and retired for the evening.

Chapter Twenty-One
RECOVERY, REDUX

"The best part about life after surgery… is life!"
—Unknown

I scrambled to see Jared as soon as visiting hours came around the next morning. When I walked into his room at 8:00 a.m., he looked awful. He looked nothing like he did when we left last night. In all honesty, he looked like he had just had the shit beat right out of him. His face was puffed up, his eyes were black and he told me that his face had been so itchy that he couldn't sleep all night.

Luckily, Dr. Bathe had just come in to see how Jared was feeling and realized he was having an allergic reaction to the pain medication. Dr. Bathe notified the anesthetist and they changed Jared's medication to fentanyl, a different type of painkiller. It took a few hours before the reaction was under control. Jared's eyes began to look better and he wasn't trying to scratch the skin off his face.

Jared looked much better on his second day of recovery. The anesthetist was in earlier that morning to check on the epidural. Jared said that he was still very sore, but we assumed that discomfort was normal after having such a major surgery. After a mere twenty-four hours of recovery, Jared made his first attempt to walk. The nurses provided him with a walker to help support his weight.

The funniest thing happened. Attempting to walk for the first time since having his stomach removed, Jared obviously wasn't moving very fast. As we slowly shuffled down the hallway, an elderly lady pushing her own walker cruises up from behind and passes by us like we're standing still. Jared looks at me and says, "Dad, I'm pathetic! She's 80 and I'm 18 years old!" I told him

147

that the more often he walked the more mobility he would have, and the easier it would be to get out of bed. Both his mother and his sister had to endure the same painful process, and I was sure that Jared could handle it.

That day Jared was able to take his first oral nourishment since surgery: ice chips. On day three Jared was still experiencing a lot of pain. The pump responsible for administering his pain medications started making beeping noises and the nurse had to call for an anesthetist. The anesthetist arrived and adjusted the dosage, which seemed to help. About one-half hour later, the pump went into alarm mode again, and the nurses had to recall the anesthetist. This time they decided to replace the pump and everything seemed kosher.

Jared began to take clear fluids, a step up from ice chips.

The following morning Jared received another visit from the anesthetist. Jared explained that the pain was getting worse again. The bed sheets were soaked. The doctor turned Jared over to check his epidural and discovered that it had almost been torn right out, was leaking all over the place, and would have to be removed. The good news was that it would be removed that day and would be replaced either with individual morphine injections or a Pain Control Pump (PCP). The PCP was the preferred option, as it would automatically infuse a controlled rate of morphine that Jared could administer himself with the push of a button. The pump would allow Jared to take a shot every 15 minutes and no more than one infusion per quarter-hour to prevent overdose. Today, Jared was able to sip consommé soup, something with a little flavour.

Finally, on day five, Jared was given a chance to taste some real food. That morning the nurse set up a tray of gelatin, Jell-o pudding, and consommé soup. Jared was doing fine with the PCP. He was walking a bit more, pushing his IV pole around the halls. As luck would have it, as Jared and I were walking around the halls, we met up with that same elderly lady, still pushing her walker. This time we stopped just long enough to say hello and she said that Jared looked better than the last time she saw him. Jared politely answered "thank you" as we walked past her.

Jared's recovery was right on schedule and by day six he was nearly ready to be discharged. He was walking around the ward two to three times a day and his pain was under control. He was eating – not much, mind you – but eating, mostly soft foods: mashed potatoes, cream soups, ice cream. On Halloween morning, the nurses removed Jared's IV and disconnected his PCP. His food tray was a smorgasbord of pudding, coffee, toast and soft-boiled eggs. The nurses had been gradually working up to his first full meal since the surgery, and after the last six days, it must have seemed like a feast.

Before lunch Dr. Mack officially discharged Jared from the hospital. We had decided that a fifty-five minute flight home would be easier on Jared than an eight-hour drive. Dr. Mack had some concerns with us flying so soon after surgery and asked us to stick around until Monday. He also wanted Jared on solids for a few more days before we left, and so did I.

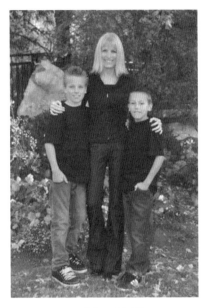

Lea and her Children

We remained at the hostel for the next three days, and it was great to have Jared with us. Jan and I went out and bought a few special things that Jared could eat, but I was paranoid that he was already eating so much and so soon after surgery. We didn't know what to expect, but I thought he would be mostly on nutritional drinks. The doctors told us, to the contrary, that Jared could eat anything he liked but he would have to eat smaller portions and eat more often. I thought about how different the simple mechanics of eating and digesting would have to be without a stomach. Essentially, Jared's stomach was now in his mouth; the digestive enzymes in Jared's saliva would have to step in and do the work of his now absent stomach. In place of having stomach acid break down his food, Jared would have to masticate his food meticulously.

Dr. Mack informed us that overall, Jared's nutritional absorption would be no different than anyone else's. His food would still pass though the duodenum and into the small bowel, he still had digestive enzymes from his pancreas and bile, which would help break down and absorb food once it found its way into the small bowel. Our family has always stayed close to the classic three-meals-a-day approach, stocking up on large amounts of food to get us through the day and to the next meal. Now we were supposed to eat smaller portions and more frequently. It would take some adjustment. Most of us were used to overeating and stuffing too much food into our stomachs at one time.

While we were still in Calgary for Jared's surgery, we had a special visit from a woman we had met through a HDGC membership web site where families affected can correspond with one another and share valuable information. Lea had been told she had the CDH1 mutation in June 2007, and her prophylactic gastrectomy had been performed at Peter Lougheed Centre in Calgary on August 20, 2007. She told us that she had been about 120 pounds before surgery and was down to about 112 pounds now. By the age of forty-one, Lea had lost her mother, a grandfather and her cousin to the disease. One uncle had been tested to be a carrier of the (CDH1) mutation. Lea believed the disease to be of her mother's ancestry.

Through her own research and speaking with others who had already travelled down that road, Lea had decided that a total gastrectomy was a doable procedure and that she would go ahead with genetic testing. Some twelve weeks later, Lea was told she had the mutation. "My boys – Alex and Garrett – were truly my biggest motivator for this whole journey," Lea told us. "I could not let them go through the pain and suffering of watching their mom die."

Genetic testing would not be available for the boys until they reach 18. By that time we all hoped there would be alternatives to the total gastrectomy, and new tests that could be performed to detect the disease earlier. Lea's visit couldn't have come at a better time. Ever since Erin's passing, communication technologies had improved so much that we had been able not only to find a lot of information on the disease, but even more importantly, we were able to find support from those who had travelled down a similar road.

The next day, Jared and I flew home while Jan drove the car back to Regina. The owner of Coles Travel had made special travel arrangements for Jared. There would be a wheelchair waiting for us at the airport and special boarding assistance. We were seated in the first row in the aircraft. Dr. Mack had voiced some concern that the flight might have adverse effects on Jared's condition, possibly excessive indigestion and nausea. Well, we were about to find out. The plane picked up speed and we were up and away. I kept a close eye on Jared throughout the entire flight and asked him if he felt any discomfort. He said he could feel it in his head but not in his stomach. I laughed, he smiled. The flight went just fine in the end, smooth and short. I think we were home before Jan had even managed to get the car out of Alberta.

Chapter Twenty-Two
HOME SWEET HOME

"As is a tale, so is life; not how long it is
but how good it is; is what matters."
—*Seneca*

We were amazed and delighted that, in the first week after his surgery, Jared was eating everything and anything, even going out to eat with his friends. We also discovered that while we were away, Kerry Joseph had been making headlines back home. On October 29th, Joseph had spoken at Erin's elementary school about the special bond he had formed with Erin. Both the school and our neighbours were helping to raise money for a special park bench in Erin's memory, which was to be placed in our neighbourhood in west Regina.

Jared, Jan and I were also invited to speak at Erin's former school. Admittedly, we were a bit of an anticlimax after the quarterback of the Riders. Nevertheless, some three hundred students and teachers gathered in the school gymnasium, and I was honoured to have the opportunity to thank everyone for all the money they had raised for Erin's memorial. The teachers had asked their students to bring in loonies and toonies, raising a total of $762.72 toward the purchase of the bench.

Things seemed to be going fine, but it wasn't long before Jared began to have problems eating. Between October 25th and December 8th Jared had lost forty-one pounds. He had dropped another ten pounds and was down to 136 pounds. Jared was now having difficulties swallowing and keeping down the food he seemed to be able to eat the previous week. I left a message with Dr. Mack in Calgary to call us. Dr. Mack mentioned it was possible Jared had a bug or an infection of some sort, but he couldn't be certain without being able to examine him in person. It was best for us to contact Dr. Malik and arrange to have Jared's blood tested and a *"barium swallow"* X-ray: an examination in which the upper gastrointestinal tract is illuminated by having the patient drink a barium solution, helping the radiologists see how the esophagus, the duodenum, and (usually) the stomach is functioning.

In the meantime, the Riders had just won the Western Division championship, beating the BC Lions 26-17. Hundreds of fans surrounded the airport until the early hours of the cool November morning to greet the team on their way back from the game. It was a big deal for Rider fans and a big deal for Saskatchewan. The Riders haven't been the most successful franchise, and it wasn't every year that we had a legitimate shot at the Grey Cup. The team had won only two Grey Cups in its history, in 1966 and 1989, and now they would represent the West on November 25ᵗʰ 2007 in the 95ᵗʰ Grey Cup in Toronto. Jared and I went along with a few of his friends to congratulate the players. We could not believe the numbers of fans that had shown up so late that night to welcome the division champs home. Jared wasn't feeling great and decided not to wander through the crowd. He waited for us to return from congratulating Mr. Joseph as he exited the airport.

Three days before the Grey Cup, the CFL awarded Kerry Joseph the award for the League's Most Outstanding Player. The day of the game came around, and the whole city was breathless with anticipation. A large contingent of boisterous riders fans would be making their way to Toronto to watch the game, but Jared, Jan and I, along with a few of Jared's friends, settled in to watch the Grey Cup on TV at home. We knew that Erin would be watching on her own big screen in the sky. We all know the result that day: Kerry Joseph fulfilled his promise to Erin. The Riders walked into the SkyDome in Toronto and beat the Winnipeg Blue Bombers in a close one, 23-19. As the camera bobbed its way through the melee of celebrating players and a hail of green and white confetti, we caught a glimpse of Joseph.

As he raised the Cup, we noticed the unmistakable bright orange I ♥ ERIN wristband dangling from Joseph's right wrist. While everyone in Saskatchewan and in pockets all around Canada were celebrating the Riders' third CFL championship, Jan and I silently lit a candle in Erin's memory. It was a Grey Cup we would never forget.

A few days after the big game, Kevin, Cheryl and their son TJ came down from Saskatoon to help us cheer the Roughriders' homecoming. We were among the thousands of fans that braved the cold weather to welcome home League MVP Kerry Joseph and the rest of the team. The local paper the next day told us that approximately 8,000 fans endured -36°C weather to welcome the Riders at Mosaic Stadium.

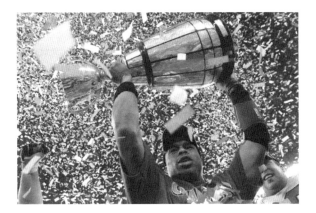

2007 League MVP Kerry Joseph

Only a few people in the stands that day would likely understand the significance of the I ♥ ERIN sign that we held as high as we could while the players streamed onto the field with the Cup, but Mr. Joseph would be one of them. Here in Saskatchewan we have some of the loudest fans in the CFL: we christened ourselves the proverbial "13th" man. Although the Riders were far from home, I believed that they still had an unfair advantage that year: Erin was their 13th man. Glen Reid, the sports broadcaster who I happened to meet at a Riders practice a few months earlier, contacted us to let us know that CBC was planning to broadcast the story behind the I ♥ ERIN wristbands.

Mr. Reid was the only media person who happened to be in the right place at the right time: he had managed to get a video of me giving Mr. Joseph and Yo Murphy their wristbands and Erin's obit inside of Mosaic Stadium. Erin's story would be a national news item. Erin's gift had a chance of being something beyond our own family. In the meantime, another of Erin's relatives – Uncle Clint, RoseMarie's brother – became the fifth family member to receive his genetic test results. Clint tested positive. This put all three of Clint's children – Summer, Caleb and Alii – at risk.

★ ★ ★

It was now December, more than a month since Jared's surgery. In that time, his recovery underwent a complete 180° reversal. He became incapable of swallowing nearly anything, and was constantly vomiting. Whatever was happening, it was getting worse. I dialed Dr. Malik's cell phone (which he had given to me in case of an emergency) and told him that Jared was beginning to waste away. He was vomiting so much that water wasn't even staying down. Dr. Malik said he would meet us at the Emergency department.

When Jared, Jan and I arrived at the hospital we told the receptionist that Dr. Malik was meeting us. She looked surprised. I told her that Jared was a special patient of his. The nurse asked about Jared's condition and we began to explain that his stomach had been removed in Calgary forty-five days prior. The receptionist had this perplexed look on her face.

The charge nurse approached and asked whether Jared had a Jejunal Loop or "Pouch" constructed in place of his stomach. We went on to explain that Jared's esophagus had been connected straight through to his duodenum via Roux-en-Y. After the nurse finally figured out what the hell Jared was talking about, we were taken directly into Emergency. They asked us so many questions that I was surprised they didn't make Jared pull up his shirt to show them his scar; but then again, I guess there aren't many people coming through Emergency without their stomach, especially at 18 years of age!

Dr. Malik must have already called Emergency to see if we had arrived, because the moment we stepped into the department, a lab technician approached us with a requisition to take a blood sample as soon as possible. Dr. Malik knew the lab results might take awhile and I guess he wanted to get the ball rolling. Dr. Malik had a look at Jared's blood test and was happy to see there were no signs of infection from the surgery. Nonetheless, Dr. Malik wanted some further tests, so Jared was admitted immediately. Dr. Malik began arranging for Jared to have his barium swallow X-ray. He told us that if his presumptions were correct, Jared was suffering from a "stricture."

A stricture, Dr. Malik explained, describes what happens when the esophagus is gradually narrowed through a build-up of scar tissue, resulting in swallowing difficulties. The body saw the Roux-en-Y as a wound and was continually trying to repair itself, thus creating a ring of scar tissue inside his esophagus. Think of it like a weld: our body is healing from the inside as well as the outside. Peptic strictures, usually due to acid reflux disease, account for seventy to eighty per cent of all esophageal strictures. But this may or may not have been the case for Jared, and we wouldn't know until after an X-ray.

It was going to be a long night. About 10:00 p.m. they found a bed on the ward. We were led to a private room. The nurses started an IV while Dr. Malik made arrangements for a dietitian to requisition a "total practical nutrition" feeding tube that would allow Jared's body to obtain nutrition intravenously. Today was Saturday, and Jared's X-ray wasn't going to be until

Monday. To make matters worse, we were told that dieticians didn't work on the weekend, which meant that the TPN feeding would also have to wait until Monday.

To prepare for the barium swallow, Jared had to drink a thick, glutinous liquid that resembled a milkshake. Apparently, the resemblance was only skin-deep.

"Dad...this tastes like SHIT. Like battery acid or something..."

"You've tasted *battery* acid?

"Well...no. But this is what battery acid tastes like, probably."

Jared could barely swallow the rest without vomiting. A female technician greeted us at the entrance to the X-ray department and led us down a semi-darkened hallway and into a room marked "Fluoroscopy-1." The tech allowed me to watch from behind a partial wall sporting a control panel and a thick pane of radiation-proof glass. From the look on her face, I was guessing that she hadn't seen many patients Jared's age with a Roux-en-Y, and I was as curious as she was to see what his surgery looked like from the inside.

The tech was totally blown away when she read Jared's chart and discovered that he had no stomach. When she asked him why, Jared told her he had inherited a genetic mutation, that he had lost both his mom and his sister to HDGC, and that he had to have a prophylactic gastrectomy to avoid the same fate. After a moment or two of stunned silence, the tech asked Jared to swallow another barium drink. A whirr and a click later, the tech thrust images of Jared's empty middle onto a set of wall mounted viewing boxes, lit from behind. We were all a bit amazed by what we saw illuminated there, in the dark.

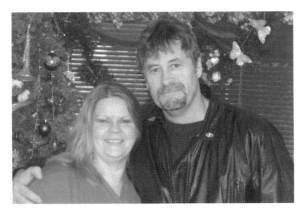

Lorie McGeough, Myself

The tech pointed to the stricture, a small protrusion about the diameter of a pea. I didn't even know what a stricture was until two days before, let alone knew what one looked like on an X-ray, but the name describes it perfectly. It's got to be one of the only medical terms that we'd come across that simply describes the thing it names. The battery-acid milkshake Jared had been forced to swallow clearly displayed the small hourglass outline of his strictured esophagus, right where they had surgically attached it to the small intestine.

After the X-ray, Jared and I returned to his room. I told him I was going downstairs to talk to Lorie, Supervisor of the GI Unit. Lorie had been there when Erin had her first scope back on May 7, 2003, and had helped my family so many times already that she had become a good friend of mine. When I arrived, the door to Lorie's office was open, and she invited me in. I told her that Jared had just finished a barium swallow, and it had revealed an esophageal stricture. I said I didn't think that Dr. Malik had even seen the radiologist's report yet, and asked her what would need to be done to fix it. Lorie said they would dilate the esophagus with a balloon, attached to an endoscope. The balloon would basically stretch out the stricture by tearing apart the hardened tissue that had formed around the inside of his esophagus. The good news, as we learned, was that the stricture was not caused by any acid reflux or gastroesophageal diseases. More importantly, the problem could be easily repaired.

Chapter Twenty-Three
STRICTURE

Dec. 10: Gastroscopy #1

Dr. Malik and Lorie quickly arranged to have Jared's stricture dilated that day. Before he could go through with the procedure, however, Dr. Malik would have to contact Dr. Mack in Calgary to update him about Jared's condition and inform him about the situation. Stricture dilation was a painful experience, even with medication. There was blood coming out of Jared's mouth and he said he felt a burning sensation in his throat after the procedure. In the evening, Jared was to begin his first TPN (total parenteral nutrition) feeding. It too looked like a milkshake, but in a big IV bag.

The nurses would have to move Jared's IV line to a much larger vein in his arm to accommodate the TPN, since it was a thicker solution than regular IV fluid, and would likely cause a small vein to collapse. About ten minutes later, Jared began to complain that his arm was becoming very sore. The nurses checked the IV site and turned down the rate of infusion. Even the new vein was having trouble accommodating the volume of TPN being administered.

It had been a very long and painful day for Jared. He was exhausted. As if he hadn't been through enough already with his surgery, now he had the stricture problem. It would have to be treated until his body surrendered and stopped trying to repair the surgical work that had been done.

Great Auntie Linda was one of the last of our relatives to receive her genetic results. She was the sixth member of the family to get tested and the second whose results came back positive for the CDH1 mutation. Her daughter, Alayne, and her son Aaron, would now have the option to be tested to find out if they are carriers of the gene.

On December 13th, Dr. Malik discharged Jared from the hospital. He had regained a total of five pounds while on TPN, which brought him up to about 141 pounds. Jared was to return for another scope in three weeks, or sooner if he began to have difficulty swallowing again. Lorie was adamant that if he had the slightest problems to give them a call. I promised her we would, but hoped everything would be fine for three weeks.

Dec. 23: Gastroscopy #2

Everything wasn't fine. I should have known not to jinx it by saying everything would be fine. Lorie was right. Jared began to stricture only fifteen days after his first procedure. It was a Sunday. I contacted Lorie at home and she got in touch with the specialist, Dr. Nel, who was on call for the weekend. Dr. Nel came over from the General Hospital to scope Jared. It was considered an emergency: we were told that Jared had strictured to the point where the endoscope wouldn't even pass through his esophagus. The upper GI scope is from 8-11mm in diameter or less than one-half inch. A normal esophagus is about 20mm. Jared's esophagus had shrunk over 12mm. No wonder he was having trouble swallowing. That night Jared was suffering from his procedure. His throat was raw and burning. His chest was sore from intermittent muscle spasms in his esophagus.

There was clearly no way to celebrate Christmas like we used to. The "festive" season felt decidedly less festive. We put up a tree, but we didn't put any gifts under it. It was our first Christmas without Erin, and Jared was now struggling to overcome complications from his own surgery. We couldn't shop or even think about exchanging presents. The people who knew, knew enough not to say Merry Christmas as we passed them on the street. Merry wasn't really in our vocabulary this year.

We did get one pleasant surprise. Erin hadn't lived to see her favourite team win the Grey Cup, so I thought it was appropriate that Jared be given the opportunity to accept the trophy on behalf of his sister. This would not have been possible if not for my good friend Ron Shatkowski and his acquaintance, Tony Playter, the Coordinator of Football Operations for the Saskatchewan Roughriders. I simply cannot put into words how special this was for us. What people have done, and continue to do, in memory of my daughter, is nothing short of extraordinary. We will never forget the look on Jared's face when the Grey Cup came through our front door. "It was quite a shock," Jared said. "When the Cup came in, I saw my sister."

On New Year's Eve, Jared was feeling well enough to go out with his friends. Jan and I had different plans: we would spend a quiet New Year's

Eve by ourselves, at home. The year 2007 was the worst year of our lives. At the stroke of midnight, Jan and I walked outside into the frozen moonlight. We could hear people yelling *"Happy New Year!"* throughout the neighbourhood. Rather than join the chorus, we shouted in our loudest voices: *F... U, 2007!*

January 3, 2008: Gastroscopy #3

Jared, Jan and I returned to the Pasqua GI Unit for the first time of the year. Jared was scheduled to have another scope/procedure. This time Dr. McHattie was the gastroenterologist who would be dilating the scar tissue in Jared's throat. It was decided that all future scopes were going to be scheduled for Thursdays with Dr. McHattie, due to the fact that Jared was now attending classes at the University of Regina and was free that day. As before, Jared suffered from the procedure. His throat was raw and his chest was sore from muscle spasms. All he could do was take a painkiller, which, ironically, had to be taken orally.

January 10, 2008: Gastroscopy #4

More blood work was needed to check Jared's B12 and iron levels. The doctors recommended that he begin a B12 injection once a month to maintain these levels, since his body could no longer absorb B12 normally without a stomach. We returned to the Pasqua GI Unit for Jared's next scope. Dr. McHattie told us that Jared would require *several* more of these procedures. I asked how many, and he said it would ultimately depend on Jared's body. Eventually the muscles in the esophagus would relax and stop trying to close.

January 17, 2008: Gastroscopy #5

We were warned about it and it had happened: we were now going to the hospital once a week. Dr. McHattie had been taking biopsies and attempting to construct a natural bridge around the stricture. The theory behind this is that each time a small biopsy is taken the body heals the tissue by forming a natural scar. Over several procedures this process would form a bridge and help to prevent the stricture from recurring. The next week(s) continued in the same vein. Other than Dr. Lewis occasionally subbing for Dr. McHattie, we fell into a torturous routine, with Jared experiencing a lot of pain during the night. By mid-February there didn't seem to be any end in sight. His body was still fighting to close his esophagus.

On February 21ˢᵗ, Dr. McHattie returned to the hospital and continued to perform biopsies that would form a natural bridge around Jared's stricture. Dr. McHattie remained completely confident that he could fix Jared up, and kept telling me not to worry. These treatments take time, every patient is different, and Jared seemed to be coming along fine. The goal was to stretch his esophagus a little more each time, until the diameter reached 20mm. Stretching too much at once would be dangerous and could result in a tear, so Dr. McHattie would have to monitor Jared's progress very carefully.

As we entered mid-March, the number of procedures went down from weekly to every two weeks, a sign that things were gradually moving in the right direction. Even two weeks apart, Jared continued to suffer from the procedure each time it was done. By trial and error, we discovered a few ways of helping Jared cope. Along with a heap of Extra Strength Tylenol and a lot of sleep, we found that drinking a cold slurpee after dilation helps reduce swelling and numbs the muscles in the esophagus, making his throat feel considerably better. Conversely, we would place heated water bottles or warm blankets on Jared's chest to help with chest pain and keep muscle spasms down.

I began to see a pattern forming, a gradual progression. It took a few weeks before Jared's next session would move to a different time slot. It was a good thing we weren't told at the beginning how many treatments to expect. I think it would have been an emotional disaster. At least this way we could take them one session at a time.

It's April now, exactly four months to the day that Jared was first treated for his stricture. On April 24ᵗʰ, it will have been six months to the day that Jared had his surgery. I wish we could say that he had made a full recovery by now, but sometimes it feels more like he's recovering from his endoscopic treatments. I am very proud of my son. He has a great deal to complain about, but never complains.

Chapter Twenty-Four

ANOTHER VISIT TO THE DOCTOR

"Success is not final, failure is not fatal:
it is the courage to continue that counts."
—Winston Churchill

In late April, we returned to Calgary to meet with Jared's surgeons, Dr. Bathe and Dr. Mack for a follow up. The doctors hadn't seen Jared for six months and he had lost a considerable amount of weight in that time.

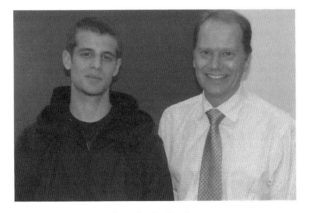

Jared, Dr. Bathe

When Dr. Bathe walked in, the first thing he said was, "Hello, skinny." The Pasqua Hospital had been forwarding Jared's medical reports so Dr. Bathe and Dr. Mack were aware of the stricture problems. After examining Jared, they could see how his scar had healed. The thickness of his scar gave some indication as to why a stricture had formed after surgery. Dr. Mack explained that not everyone develops a "hypertrophic" scar (the thickening of a scar that follows the outline of a wound). The condition was generally thought to be more common in Eastern countries such as China and in people with a darker skin pigment. Nonetheless, the doctors were both pleased with Jared's overall progress. Though he had lost weight, his body mass index was fine and the doctors told Jared that he should expect to regain half of his weight back. I hoped they were right.

It was a very long six months before Jared began to feel even remotely normal again. He said he had almost forgotten what it felt like to not feel sick. Jared struggled with indigestion and nausea every time he ate and the only time he felt decent was when he wasn't eating. Since he had to eat every two hours, he didn't feel decent most of the time. The doctors weren't kidding or cutting Jared any slack when they told us that full recovery would take up to a year.

I felt disgusted watching Jared suffer through the surgery, but the stricture was something that really made things worse than they had to be. Not once did Jared complain about how he felt. Once he said, "I really miss my stomach, Dad" – but we both knew that was nothing in comparison to what Erin had suffered. Jared had managed to get the surgery that Erin wanted and needed but couldn't have. We flew back to Regina that same day. The doctors told us that if Jared was doing well, they would like to see him again in one year's time.

★ ★ ★

The first week of February we were back. Jared was going into his seventh gastroscopy, we learned that another one of Erin's relatives had received news concerning her genetic testing. Erin's 19-year-old cousin, Summer, tested positive for the CDH1 mutation. Summer had inherited the genetic mutation from her father, Clinton, RoseMarie's brother. Because of her age, Summer was already considered high risk: she had an eighty-three per cent chance of developing the disease, as well as a forty per cent chance of developing lobular breast cancer. Even more devastating was the further discovery that Summer was four months pregnant.

Summer began consultations with Dr. Bathe regarding her options for surgery and the risks that would be involved. Summer was confronted with something akin to Sophie's Choice: either her stomach would be removed right away and she might lose her baby, or she wait until after the baby is born, knowing that the disease could be passed on genetically. She decided to take her chances that the child might be born without becoming a carrier. She said she wanted to be a mom so bad and wonders if she's being selfish. We don't know. As much as we now know we just don't know anything. Our breath is, again, collectively held. Only time will tell.

★ ★ ★

On May 1st Jared had his fifteenth gastroscopy. It had been three weeks since the last procedure, which meant things were finally starting to improve. When we walked through all the familiar doors of the GI Unit it felt like we had come back from a long holiday. That was a good feeling. The next one wouldn't be until June 5th, thirty-five days later. Dr. McHattie turned out to be right: things were improving in their own time. In mid-June I was honoured when Erin's elementary school – St. Josaphat – let me know they wanted to do something special to honour Erin's memory. We agreed to establish a special award in Erin's name and the result was the *I LOVE ERIN* Award. The award would be given annually to a student who met the following criteria:

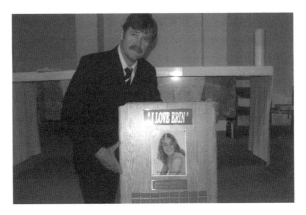

Myself - I LOVE ERIN Award

1. He/she would have to be elected by his/her fellow Grade Eight students.

2. The teachers must approve the candidate.

3. The award is *not* to be based on academics or community service.

4. He/she must be trustworthy and demonstrate a compassion for other people.

Since I was sponsoring the award, I managed to convince the school that the prize would be a gift of my choice, with no restrictions. Winner of the annual *I LOVE ERIN* award receive a new laptop computer. Jan also established a bursary, the *Erin Lawrence Memorial Award*, through Erin's former high school. As with the elementary students, we set out four criteria the winning student would have to meet in order to receive the award:

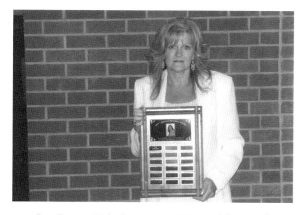

Jan Reap - Erin Lawrence Memorial Award

1. He/she would have to be elected by his/her fellow Grade Twelve students.

2. The teachers must approve the candidate.

3. The award is not to be based on academics or community services.

4. He/she must be trustworthy and demonstrate a compassion for other people.

The winner of the high school award would receive five hundred dollars cash.

In early July, Jared and I decided it was time to go back to Amisk Lake. It was much earlier in the year than our usual trips, but we were told that the Walleye fishing was supposed to be good. We drove six hours to Amisk for a four-day trip. Unlike last time, the weather was beautiful. It was so hot on the second day that we used an entire tube of sun block and still managed to burn. Last time we were there, we couldn't eat a shore lunch because of all the rain, but this time we were fortunate to have both great fishing and fantastic weather and managed to get in two lunches.

We caught our limit in Northern Pike and Walleye in just three days. I must admit Jared was a better fisherman than I was on that trip. He was having all the luck: the Walleye seemed to be swimming over themselves to get hooked on his worm harness. Sometimes he couldn't get the line back in the water fast enough to catch another one. I thought we would have to fish the full three days to catch our limit, but instead we had to leave a day early.

In late July, Jared had his seventeenth gastroscopy. It had been fifty-three days since the last procedure. Dr. McHattie remained confident that Jared would continue to improve. At that point, more emphasis would be on blood work rather than the stricture. It had been seven months since Jared was first diagnosed with a stricture, and we had come a long way since the gauntlet of weekly procedures. Things were finally beginning to return to normal, or at least, a new normal was beginning to establish itself.

Since Erin had passed away, Jared's life had been a constant series of mental and physical challenges. He had to deal with finding out he, too, inherited the CDH1 mutation, he was facing a one to two per cent mortality rate after having his stomach totally removed to (presumably) eliminate the risk of developing HDGC, and finally he had to confront the difficulties of esophageal stricture and the equally difficult and painful process of dilation. That's a lot of hurt to process, but he never complained...

Chapter Twenty-Five
A BIRTHDAY MEMORIAL / VACATION 2008

"You can't change the past but you can ruin the present
by worrying over the future."
—Walt Kennedy

It would have been Erin's 22nd birthday. Friends and neighbours moved through a small playground on the west end of the city, a few blocks from our house, as if there was going to be a party. The gathering was, in fact, the dedication ceremony for a park bench named in Erin's memory. The idea for the bench was the brainchild of two neighbours, Loretta Froh and Bonnie Gorski. They established a registered fundraiser with the City and generated over $3,000 through private donations and the support of both Erin's elementary and high schools. The elementary fundraiser featured Kerry Joseph as a guest speaker, who told the students about how he had met Erin, and the special friendship he had formed with the former St. Josaphat student. He talked about the importance of living bravely. We wore special white I ♥ ERIN t-shirts to commemorate the occasion.

As we made our way around the small thicket of pine trees cresting the hill of the park, we were suddenly overwhelmed with people. I had only expected a handful of friends and relatives, but *everyone* showed up. Not just friends and relatives, but friends of friends, neighbours, even people who lived in the neighbourhood that we didn't really know. I counted over fifty people, all there to honour Erin's memory. Jan's sister had scheduled her annual visit from B.C. to coincide with the dedication, and Erin's Aunt Mel and her family had made the 2-1/2 half hour trek from Rocanville. A few of Erin's girlfriends wore their Roughriders gear, knowing it's what their Chief would have wanted.

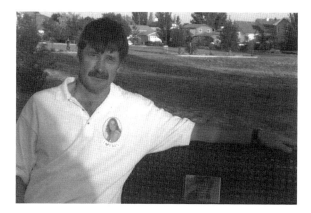

Myself -Erin's Bench

A few weeks later, we decided we would go on our first family vacation since losing Erin. We returned to our favourite destination: Orlando. It wasn't the same without Erin, nothing ever will be. We were still in the process of trying to see things clearly through the lens of the new normal. Grieving is a strange thing. Everything in the world takes on a slightly different inflection, because you're constantly made aware there is something missing from it. The new normal is disorienting at first: it means reconstructing your relationships not only with people, but with places and things.

We made the loop through Disney World's various theme parks. Jared and I made sure to hit our favourite rides in honour of "Chief." It was early September and the parks were practically dead. Most kids were already back in school and hurricane season was about to begin. For the most part, the weather was intensely hot and never dropped below 90°F or 32.3°C during the day. The only time it cooled down was when "Hurricane Ike" swept through the Gulf Coast and treated us to an old-fashioned electrical storm. The pools at the hotel were completely empty, except for us. We got a giddy thrill at hearing the sounds of our own voices echoing through empty space and feeling the sharp razor-chill of a distant but approaching storm. Somehow, it just felt great.

Despite the looming threat of the storm, we decided we would make the most of our final day in Florida and decided to stop at a local flea market in Kissimmee. Sure enough, as we made our way towards the salmon pink deco-style building, the sky opened up. Quickly taking shelter from the weather, we ran into the flea market and almost smack into the booth of an artist who specialized in airbrushing. After showing the artist both an I ♥ ERIN wristband and the Riders' logo, I asked him if he could synthesize the two to create a personalized logo. About twenty minutes later, we were handed a t-shirt, emblazoned with a perfect replica of the Riders' trademark green, white, and black "S", encircled by the familiar bright orange wristband, at once bringing together Erin's great love of football, and our great love for Erin.

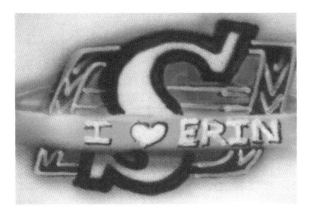

Personalized Logo

The final leg of our vacation involved traveling to British Columbia. It was a long flight: we flew directly from Orlando to Toronto, and then we had to clear customs and fly another 4-1/2 hours to get to B.C. We landed on the 11th of September at Vancouver International Airport. After we arrived, I rented a vehicle and we stayed a few days with Jan's sister, Bonnie. Jared, Jan and I made arrangements to meet with Dr. Huntsman, the genetic pathologist who developed the blood test to screen for the CDH1 mutation, while we were in town.

We knew it would be something of an experience to meet Dr. Huntsman in person after months of correspondence by e-mail. It was because of his research and dedication that Jared had his surgery. I thought the two would like to meet. Putting things in perspective, I would have to say our meeting with Dr. Huntsman was a bittersweet experience. I believe we both had something to offer each other. As one of Dr. Huntsman's associates told me, it was unusual for them to meet the families affected by their own genetic tests: they test hundreds of samples worldwide and usually never get a chance to meet the families. Despite this, Dr. Huntsman and his researchers were always acutely aware that every sample has a face, every face has a name, and every name has a family.

Dr. Huntsman had taken time out of his busy day to sit down with us for a few hours. We discussed Erin, the CDH1 mutation, and the circumstances that led Dr. Huntsman to pursue his research into Hereditary Diffuse Gastric Cancer. If not for this research in HDGC or his work in isolating the CDH1 mutation, Jared wouldn't even have discovered that he was a carrier of the gene to this day. Dr. Huntsman talked a little bit about the history of this disease. He talked about Napoleon Bonaparte. There were hints that Napoleon had passed away from HDGC: the diminutive would-be emperor's family had had a strong history of cancer, and it has been suggested by some medical historians that he had in fact suffered from stomach cancer.

Dr. Huntsman also told us there are some families that have been tested and linked to having this mutation going back four or five, even six or seven, generations. I asked if that would make them distant relatives of ours, to which Dr. Huntsman smiled and said, no, each family has a unique 'spelling mistake' in their DNA chain that determines whether or not they are genetically related. If the spelling mistake is found to be in the same location as the DNA being tested, then they would be presumed to be a relative.

The reverse is true if a DNA sample is determined to have the same spelling mistake that would make them a relative. This is how they are able to genetically track generations of this disease. In very rare circumstances, this is not the case: DNA spelling mistakes can be replicated and not be related. Occasionally, Dr. Huntsman told us, they had discovered the 'replica' of a mutated gene to be a non-relative. Today, there are over one hundred families that have been found to be carriers of CDH1.

It was a pleasure finally meeting face-to-face with Dr. Huntsman and his team. As we were leaving Dr. Huntsman's office, he asked if he could have five I ♥ ERIN wristbands. I was honoured to oblige. It was at that moment I realized that Dr. Huntsman was another one of the many people who Erin had inspired. While spending time in B.C., we couldn't pass up the opportunity to support our Roughriders, who were in Vancouver for a game against the Lions. We managed to swing some tickets, compliments of Jan's nephew Dion. For those of you unfamiliar with the Riders, there's one thing I can tell you, Rider fans are well-known as some of the most rabid fans in the Canadian Football League. I'm always amazed that the Riders seem to have a fan base no matter where they happen to be playing. We lost the game, but it was a good feeling to be part of the hundreds of fans that showed their support that night for their Green and White.

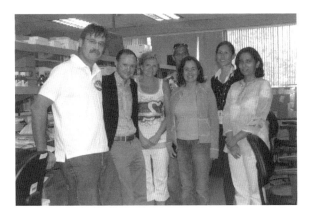

Myself, Dr. Huntsman, Jan, Jared, Dr. Huntsman Team

We returned home from our vacation in the first week of October and things slowed down a bit. Jared was scheduled for another round of routine blood work to monitor his B12 levels. Normally, our stomach lining secretes an "intrinsic factor" that helps absorb vitamin B12, a vitamin essential for growth. This was exactly the reason why Dr. Huntsman asked Jared how tall he was before the surgery. After his stomach was removed, he would effectively stop growing: *"rather be short and alive than tall and dead."* This is why Jared would need a B12 supplement. Our bodies can never have too much B12 stored in the blood. Any excess is usually dispensed through urination. The normal range of Vitamin B12 in the body is between 200-900 "picograms" per milliliter (pg/ml). Anything under 200 is considered to be a deficiency and can lead to Pernicious Anemia.

It wasn't until Halloween, a year after Jared's discharge from the hospital, that Jared went in for another gastroscopy with Dr. McHattie; a full ninety-five days since his last procedure. In that time he'd gained about five pounds and was now up to a relatively healthy 140 pounds. Before going in for the procedure, Jared elected *not* to be put under any kind of painkiller; he wanted to go cold turkey. Since he had been through so many of these damn things already, this would be number eighteen, Jared decided that he might be able to manage. The nurses all commended him for his courage, especially our old friend, nurse Mardel. She was very proud of him, and so was his dad.

Jared's B12 levels were constantly dropping, so Dr. McHattie wanted to make sure that we kept them in the normal range. Jared had to increase his B12 injections from monthly to daily for one week, once a week for six weeks, and then finally once a month for a full year.

This isn't going to be temporary: without a stomach, Jared will require B12 injections for the rest of his life. He will constantly have to be monitored in order to maintain anything like the 'norm' for his age and diet. But normal is anything but, these days.

CODA: Summer's Choice

Summer asks us, the world, if she's being selfish. I don't know how to answer her, I don't think anyone does. She knows the odds aren't good: 70/30 in favour of the disease, we're told. She knows the risk she is taking. It will be done, but not yet, because there is life there; Summer is four months pregnant at the time. The television news anchor calls it a genetic time bomb. Behind him, red and blue strands of DNA show us the calligraphy of an entire history: hers, ours. A woman's voice, unseen, says 'not yet.'

Summer moves across the screen, arms bare, carrying a blue tin of instant coffee. They probably told her to do something normal, something she does everyday, like the camera isn't even there. There are flowers on the table. She takes a deep breath and tells us she wishes she didn't know. Knowing makes it harder because it means having to make a choice, not only about her own life, but the life of her child. Is it selfish to want to love, to want to be a mom, even though it could mean passing on the disease?

She tells us, the world, that she's decided to take the chance. She will name her Mikka. It's Hebrew, and it means gift from God.

CONCLUSIONS

Hereditary Diffuse Gastric Cancer. What is it? I know what it is for me, I know exactly how to answer that question, even though I'm no doctor. It's a killer. HDGC swept two people from my life before I even knew what it was, before I knew that it even existed. It is my hope this book will help educate others and promote awareness of HDGC. We often find out about things today that we wish we were aware of yesterday. My father used to have a saying: there's no use closing the barn door after the horse runs out. When RoseMarie passed away, this HDGC wasn't known to be hereditary. I wish, and that word hardly describes it, that we had known the disease was hereditary before we lost Erin.

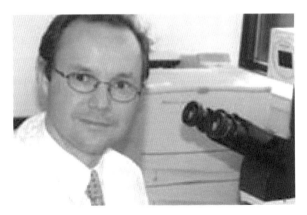

Dr. Huntsman

Since the gene was discovered in 1998, Dr. Huntsman's research in HDGC in 2005 has given humankind the opportunity to have a blood test to determine who has inherited the disease. Unfortunately, someone has to be affected by this disease before their blood can be screened. DNA has to be extracted from the blood in order to isolate the particular spelling mistake in a person's DNA string that would identify them as a carrier. Once screened and found to have the mutation, other family members or any relative can have a simple blood test to determine if they are a carrier of the CDH1 mutation.

We hope Dr. Huntsman will continue his research in this area, and someday develop a test to diagnose this disease in its earliest stages. By doing this, it would help in the prevention of unnecessary prophylactic gastrectomies. As of 2014, we still do not have an accurate screening process for HDGC, only diagnostic tools. Endoscopies can take biopsies of the stomach. Special contrast ultrasounds can measure the thickness of the stomach wall. But in most cases, the disease is usually well advanced before a person has become symptomatic.

You might be asking yourself: what are some of the symptoms? How do I know if I have this type of cancer? I can only tell you from my experience that the disease is capable of masking itself very well. The first symptom is usually something minor, like indigestion or a constant feeling of being "full." The problem is that these symptoms are so common they usually don't raise any red flags with doctors. Indigestion is not a killer and there are a lot of people with stomach problems of various kinds. My advice is that you insist on taking your health into your own hands. Ask to see a specialist, especially if there is a history of stomach cancer or stomach problems in your family.

You're a long time dead. Apologies and regrets for missed opportunities do not bring our loved ones back. I can only blame myself for not being more aggressive with my family's health. Ignorance is not an excuse. The Internet now places a world of knowledge at our fingertips. I only wish I knew then what I know now about HDGC. It is for this reason that I have written this book and chosen to share my story. I hope the reader will have gained a clearer understanding of the disease. The appendices that follow provide even more information about where to get help, what to look for, and some options that are available. Maybe somewhere, someday, this information could help save someone's life.

When RoseMarie passed away in 1991, almost nothing was known or published about HDGC. We weren't deceived. What we were told was based on what was then known about stomach cancer. It was not properly diagnosed until 1998, when it was identified to be hereditary. Education is a big part of tracking this disease. Unfortunately, you must be aware that it's in your family tree. It can lay dormant for generations and then passed on without affecting your life and you don't even know you're a carrier. You, a family member or a relative can be a carrier. Traditionally it affects people age thirty-eight plus, but for reasons unknown today, it is now being found in people much younger.

Erin was the youngest person in North America, at twenty years old, known to pass away from HDGC. The disease is killing our children. I want to stop it from destroying other families. The only way something will change is to do something about it. I cannot bring my family back or change the facts. This disease is in Canada and various other places in the world, and it seems to be getting stronger. In 2007, only eighty documented families were known to have Hereditary Diffuse Gastric Cancer. In 2008, it was found that over one hundred families had the disease. Some of Erin's relatives live in Saskatchewan, but there are others we don't know about, where they live, or who they are. We were too late for one of them already: last year Jan and I attended a funeral service for one of Erin's young cousins. We never knew her personally or anything about her condition until we read her obituary. HDGC is surfacing and killing our children. Let's stop it by catching up to it, by identifying carriers from the outset and not be relegated to following a trail of destruction.

My daughter was told it was too late and she could not be helped. However, Erin was able to give her family and relatives a *gift*. Her sacrifice has allowed for DNA screening tests to identify other carriers of the CDH1 mutation in her family and her relatives. The dividends are paying off: two of Erin's great uncles were both tested for the mutation in the latter part of 2007, and neither of them carries the mutation. If we look at one branch of the family tree, beginning with the ancestors, we know that Erin's great-great-grandfather Donald passed away from stomach cancer and passed the mutation down to his son Gordon. Gordon had five children, one passing away in infancy, and of the four remaining children two were carriers of the mutation. One of the carriers was Gordon's daughter, Linda. Linda has one daughter and one grandson. At the time of writing, both have elected not to be tested. I hope this doesn't prove to be a mistake for their family. Margaret, RoseMarie's mother, had five children. RoseMarie passed away from the disease. Our daughter, Erin passed away from the disease. Margaret's son, Clinton has tested positive as a carrier of the CDH1 mutation. The other three children tested negative. Clinton has three children. His oldest daughter, Summer, has tested positive for the mutation. Alii has tested positive for the mutation and elected to have surgery. Caleb tested negative for the mutation.

We can now see how RoseMarie inherited the mutation. If we use fifty per cent as a ratio and round up, three dependents have a chance of inheriting the mutation. RoseMarie and I had two children. I understand *how* it was possible for the gene to be passed on to Erin. What I don't understand is *why* both of my children, *one hundred per cent*, of my family managed to inherit this genetic mutation. When I asked Dr. Huntsman the same question, he just shrugged his shoulders and said we were unlucky. His answer brought me back to terrifying thoughts about the randomness of things. No matter how probable something could be, nothing is ever certain. A DNA sequence that contains instructions to make a protein is known as a gene. The complete genome for a human contains about 20,000 genes on 23 pairs of chromosomes. RoseMarie had both a good copy and a bad copy of this gene, this gives a fifty per cent chance of passing this mutation on to her children.

You have to accept changes in life, you have to accept pain, or you cannot accept life, because life is change, and change is often painful. All sorts of randomness actually turned out in our favour: I think of the fortuitous moment in which Dr. Malik and Dr. Bathe happened to call at the same moment and the day that a gastroenterologist by the name of Dr. Debra Wirtzfield happened to be giving a seminar on **Hereditary Diffuse Gastric Cancer** in the same hospital Jared was having his surgery. Most importantly, although Erin didn't live long enough to see it, she saved her brother's life, and opened the possibility of saving many others.

The French philosopher Blaise Pascal once described faith as a gift. What I think he meant was that a gift, a pure act of selfless giving, was something that could not be understood from within the limits of human reason. Of all the phrases or quotes used in this book, the one listed below best encapsulates my own philosophy of life. It doesn't come from Pascal, or any other philosopher for that matter. I didn't find it in one of the great books of Western Civilization. Rather, I found it in our local newspaper. It was spoken by Erin's friend, Mr. Kerry Joseph:

"It's not meant for us to understand in this lifetime."
—*Kerry Joseph*

"It's been said, time heals all wounds. I do not agree. The wounds remain. In time, the mind, protecting its sanity, covers them with scar tissue and the pain lessens. But it is never gone."
—*Rose Kennedy*

SPECIAL THANKS

Words cannot adequately express my gratitude to all of the people who came into our lives and showed their support and compassion for my family and me. I pray this will never happen again to anyone else, but that would be nothing short of a miracle! I hope Dr. Huntsman will continue his research in HDGC and some day that medical science will develop a preventative test for the disease. I thank all the doctors.

We never took "No" for an answer. Sometimes it just wasn't in my vocabulary. At the very beginning of our troubles, a doctor told me that for strong cancer you needed strong medicine. I can now honestly say that for aggressive cancer, you need aggressive action! I can't say enough about the people who helped us through it all. Since I lost both my first wife and our daughter, I've come to learn that life is a gift. Words cannot express my loss. Parts of me are dead. But others have come alive. The person I wish to thank the most is Erin herself. With her sacrifice, she gave the ultimate gift to her family. I want to thank her for saving her brother's life, and for making me a better person.

★ ★ ★

I also want to specifically thank the following individuals:

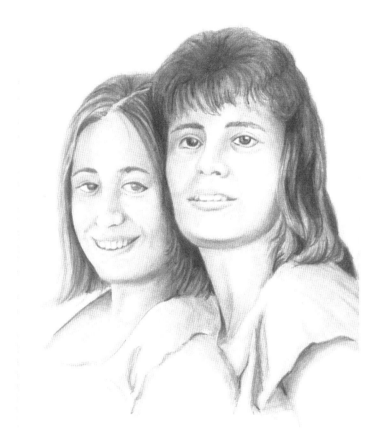

Artist Composition of Erin 13 yrs of age with her mother RoseMarie

RoseMarie Lawrence and **Erin Lawrence**
"Life is not measured by the breaths we take, but by the moments that take our breath away."

CARE GIVERS: Donna and Owen Sarauer, Lyn and Grant Schmidt, Cheryl Hack, Kimberly Werschler.

CO-OP: Ashley, Blair, Brad, Brett, Brianne, Carol, Clara, Dayle, Dejana, Denise M., Denise W., Dianne, Jeannette, Jennifer, Jennifer Gibson, Joanne, Jocelynn, Judy, Karla, Kathy, Keith D., Kelsey, Kent, Linda, Lonnie, Marcie, Pam, Pat, Ron, Sam B., Sarah B., Sean, Shane, Stewart, Sylvia, Troy, Wendy, Val Smith, Wayne.

DOCTORS: Dr. I. Y. Aboo, Dr. O. F. Bathe, Dr. J.W. Carter, Dr. P. Gorman, Dr. J. C. Hubbard, Dr. D. Huntsman, Dr. E. Lemire, Dr. W. Lewis, Dr. Lynch, Dr. L. Mack, Dr. R. A. Malik, Dr. J. D. McHattie, Dr. J.S. McMillan, Dr. Del a Ray Nel, Dr. Salim

Genetic Counselor: Katherine Osczevski

ERIN'S FRIENDS: Ashley Balysky, Bri Bast, Courtney Braaten, Aaron Bourassa, Mike Chambers, Tyler Daku, Mya Demchuk, Christine Eckel, Tricia Fluter, Jen Gibson, Tyler Guillemen, Vincenzo Grenello, Chandi Hack, Andy Hilderman, Brittany Hoffman, Dallas Hordichuk, Joe Johnston, Kyle Kapell, Rylan Kozey, Lisa Kuyek, Sara Lake, Tyler Lane, Mike Landry, Lisa Luzny, Kyle Mader, Lindsay Miller, Megan Mohr, Devin Morrisette, Josh Patterson, Shawn Pederson, Corey Pielak, Lindsay Prystupa, Ali Pulvermacher, Sean Reynolds, Jordan Sanders, Nicole Sarauer, Brett Schmidt, Merlin Sinclair, Jesse James Stewart, Nathan Wolbaum, Orlanda Wilchuk, Jacinta Wingerter, Amanda Wolfe.

FRIENDS AND NEIGHBOURS: Shelley and Wayne Cole, Dion Greene, Bonnie Gorski, Bonnie Greene, Loretta Froh, Kirby and Natalie Kazael, Terry Saen, Jackie and Bob Mason

SPECIAL PEOPLE: All of the relatives who put Erin first in their lives.
Brett Schmidt (boyfriend) for always being there for Erin
Edwin and Louella Fesser for all their spiritual guidance and support.
Ron Shatkowski and Tony Playter for bringing the Grey Cup into our residence and presenting it to Jared Lawrence.
Mr. Kerry Joseph for his compassion and kindness.
CBC Sports journalist Glenn Reid and Regina Leader-Post Sports Columnist Rob Vanstone for their articles.
Janet Reap and Riffel High School for helping to create the
Erin Lawrence Memorial Bursary
Karen Humphrey for out of province accommodations
Lea Trenholm for her testimonial and support

Lorie McGeough for her personal and 24hr. professional support

Teachers and students of St. Josaphat School, neighbours and friends for their contribution to Erin's Bench

Special thanks to Mr. Fuchs for helping to create the "I Love Erin" Award at St. Josaphat School

Andy, April, Diane, Gail, Olivia, Shannon and all the nurses who work on Ward 3B at the Pasqua Hospital

Everyone at the Allan Blair Cancer Centre for their compassionate care for Erin.

REFERENCES

I wish to acknowledge the following websites, which provided invaluable research materials that helped us over the course of our journey and in the preparation of this book:

Cotton, P.B. & Williams, C.B. (1996) "Basic Endoscopic Equipment" in Practical Gastrointestinal Endoscopy, 4th ed. Blackwell Publishers. www.blackwellpublishing.com/xml/dtds/4-0/help/10003420_chapter_1.pdf. Accessed June 1, 2014.

Mukherjee, S. "Esophageal Stricture" on Medscape: http://emedicine.medscape.com/article/175098-overview. Accessed June 1, 2014.

Native American Cancer Research Organization http://natamcancer.org/page136.html. Accessed June 1, 2014.

No Stomach for Cancer www.nostomachforcancer.org/gastric-cancer/hereditary-diffuse-gastric-cancer. Accessed June 1, 2014.

Stanford University, Genetics Counseling http://cancer.stanfordhospital.com/forpatients/services/geneticcounseling/hdgc. Accessed June 1, 2014.

Yahoo. Hereditary Diffuse Cancer Group http://health.groups.yahoo.com/group/HDGC/ membership site. Accessed June 1, 2014. http://groups.yahoo.com/group/HDGC/files/TG.pdf (Members only)

Young Adult Cancer: www.youngadultcancer.ca/. Accessed June 1, 2014.

Appendix A
INFORMATION ON HDGC

Some informative articles about Hereditary Diffuse Gastric Cancer can be obtained through numerous sources. Below are some choice quotations from several of these sources, which were chosen to help facilitate some of the questions and concerns of readers that want to know more about this disease.

"HDGC is believed to have existed since the time of Napoleon Bonaparte. The CDH1 gene was first found to be a hereditary risk factor for gastric cancer in 1998… The average age for someone with HDGC to be diagnosed with gastric cancer is 38. Women with HDGC also have an increased risk of lobular breast cancer."[2]

★ ★ ★

"HDGC is a genetic condition. This means that the cancer risk and other features of HDGC can be passed from generation to generation in a family."[3]

★ ★ ★

---

2 http://erinsgift.ca/hdgc-hereditary-diffuse-gastric-cancer/. Accessed June 1, 2014.
3 Ibid.

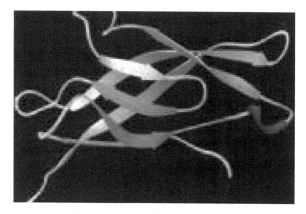

Caption: E-cadherin Protein

"The average age of onset of gastric cancer in HDGC is 38 years old, with individuals as young as 14 having been diagnosed. The estimated lifetime risk of developing gastric cancer by age 80 is 67% for men and 83% for women."

"Mutations in the E-cadherin (CDH1) gene have been identified in SOME families with this syndrome and genetic testing is now available. However, CDH1 mutations cause only 1-3% of all gastric cancers and in families with a strong history of diffuse gastric cancer, only one-third to one-half are due to CDH1 mutations."[4]

* * *

"Normally, every cell has two copies of each gene; one inherited from the mother and one inherited from the father. HDGC has an autosomal dominant inheritance pattern, in which a mutation happens in only one copy of the gene. This means a parent with a gene mutation may pass along a copy of their normal gene or a copy of the gene with the mutation. Therefore, a child who has a parent with a mutation has a 50% chance of inheriting that mutation. A brother, sister or parent of a person who has a mutation also has a 50% chance of having the same mutation."[5]

4 Stanford University, Genetics Counselling: http://cancer.stanford.edu/patient_care/services/geneticCounseling/HDGC.html. Accessed June
5 Ibid.

* * *

"Unfortunately, an endoscope every 6-12 months with biopsies is <u>not</u> an effective diagnostic tool [for HDGC]. A patient can undergo a 'high-magnification endoscopy with methylene blue chromoscopy, endoscopic ultrasonography, CT and PET scans.' New techniques for diagnosing diffuse gastric cancer are under investigation but none have been proven effective in <u>early</u> detection at this time . . . . Prophylactic gastrectomy is the only reliable preventive treatment for patients with CDH1 gene mutations. Not every CDH1 carrier will develop gastric cancer. A patient who carries a CDH1 mutation has a 50% chance of passing on the mutation to each of their children. Testing children younger than 18 is generally not recommended. The youngest recorded patient diagnosed with HDGC was 14... Patients seriously considering prophylactic gastrectomy should make sure their surgeon is well experienced in this procedure and is knowledgeable about HDGC risks to ensure that the *best* technique is chosen while minimizing the risk of surgical complications... The decision to carry out a prophylactic gastrectomy must consider the +1% risk of death associated with the procedure and nearly 100% risk of long term complications including infection, leakage at the surgery site as well as the fact that not every CDH1 carrier will develop gastric cancer."[6]

* * *

"Prophylactic gastrectomy is a major surgical procedure associated with predictable morbidity and potential mortality rates and thus should only be performed by expert surgeons after counseling by geneticists, dieticians, and gastroenterologists."[7]

Surgical Procedure
Jejunal Loop Fistula Roux-en-Y Jejunol with jejuno-jejunostomy Fistula[8]

***

www.youngadultcancer.ca is a website designed specifically for young people who have cancer or have supported someone suffering from cancer.

6 Information cited from website active at an earlier time that can no longer be validated.
7 Information cited from website active at an earlier time that can no longer be validated.
8 H. William Scott, Jr., Michael G. Weidner. Ann Surg. 1956 May; 143(5): 682–695. www.pubmedcentral.nih.gov/articlerender.fcgi?artid=1465240. Accessed June 1, 2014.

The site is especially useful, since many existing support groups simply are not designed to address health and social issues particular to young adults, which are, of course, very different from those that affect someone that is fifty or seventy.

Appendix B

FAMILIES

"Founder and Recurrent CDH1 Mutations in Families with Hereditary Diffuse Gastric Cancer"[9]

Published in the June 6, 2007 issue of the *Journal of the American Medical Association* and written with the collaboration of forty M.D.'s, PhD's, and MSc's (including our Dr. Huntsman), the stated objective of the study was "to determine whether recurring germline *CDH1* mutations occurred due to independent mutational events or common ancestry." The study goes on to say that researchers in Austria "first identified" the gene in three Maori families in New Zealand, and that "the youngest reported death from HDGC was in a 16-year-old adolescent from the Maori Family in which the first *CDH1* germline mutations were described" (2368). The largest CDH1 germline mutation affected family found in Canada is the Bradfield Family in Newfoundland: "the incidence of mortality from gastric cancer in Newfoundland is the highest in Canada at 1.7 times the Canadian average. Within Newfoundland, the regions his family comes from (Avalon Peninsula and southeast coast) are the highest-risk areas within the province" (2370).

★ ★ ★

SUTHERLAND FAMILY TREE

More detailed and updated information on the Sutherland family tree can be found at: http://erinsgift.ca/sutherland-family-tree/. Please feel free to add your comments or questions on the website regarding genetic information or relatives affected by the CDH1 mutation. Carriers of the CDH1 mutation in the genealogy below are indicated in bold face.

9 JAMA. 2007;297(21):2360-2372. doi:10.1001/jama.297.21.2360.

- **Donald Sutherland**, born 1863 Caithness Scotland, married Margaret Hamilton. Donald immigrated to Whitby, Ontario, Canada in 1883 and arrived in Saskatchewan in the spring of 1896. His wife and family joined him in the fall of the same year. They had a total of eight children: Donaldina, John, James, Amelia, Angus, Janet, **Gordon**, and Henry. Donald passed away from stomach cancer in 1910.

- **Gordon Sutherland,** born Feb. 19 1897 married Elizabeth Brown, who died due to complications from childbirth in 1928. Gordon remarried Francis Coghill in 1935. They had four children: Henry (1936), **Margaret** (1939), Earl (1942), and **Linda** (1947).

- **Linda** had one child, Alayne (1972). As of August 2009, Alayne has elected to forego genetic testing. Alayne also has one child, Aaron (1987), who has also chosen not to be tested for the disease (as of August 2009).

- **Margaret Sutherland** married Ray Birkenshaw and had five children: Cindy (1960), **RoseMarie** (1961), Melodie (1963), **Clinton** (1965), and Adam (1983).

- **RoseMarie** Birkenshaw married Luke Lawrence. We had two children: **Erin** (1986) and **Jared** (1989). RoseMarie passed away January 7, 1991, and **Erin** on August 6, 2007 at twenty years of age. **Jared** genetically tested positive as a carrier of the CDH1 mutation, and had a prophylactic gastrectomy in 2007.

- **Clinton** has had three children: **Summer** (1988), **Alii** (1991), and Caleb (1992). Summer tested positive as a carrier of the CDH1 mutation, as of 2014 she is still contemplating having surgery.

- **Summer** has two children Mikka (2009), and Harlow (2013) who have not been tested due to age.

- **Alii** tested positive as a carrier of the CDH1 mutation and had a prophylactic gastrectomy in 2014. "Erin's Gift" ultimately saved her life. Pathology reports *confirmed* that Alii's stomach was in the early stages of the disease.

★ ★ ★

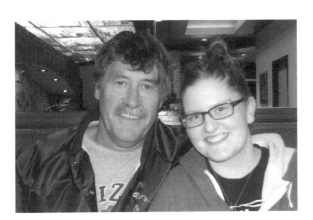

Myself, Alii-Birkenshaw-Morson

TESTIMONIAL
ALII BIRKENSHAW–MORSON

"After finding out at 21 years of age that I carry the CDH1 gene I decided to go ahead and have my stomach removed just to be on the safe side.

On March 13, 2014 my life was changed forever. After a week in the hospital I went home to Red Deer to stay with my mom. My three week appointment was April 9, 2014 I was feeling good and anxious all at the same time knowing I was going to get my pathology report. Dr. Bathe told me they found some cancer cells in my stomach. Just hearing the word cancer gives me chills but to hear someone tell you that cancer had started in your body is something I will never forget.

That day in the clinic and the day of surgery all I could feel was Erin's presence no way someone could be as calm as I was without Erin's help.

I will always be thankful to Erin for 'Erin's Gift' without it who knows where I would have been in just a few short months."

—*Alii Birkenshaw-Morson*

The Sutherland Family tree listed above is only one branch of the descendants of Donald and Margaret Sutherland. Where the disease has surfaced, fifty per cent of these descendants have tested positive to be a carrier of the CDH1 mutation, and two people have passed away. It is my hope that some day we can stop the spread of this genetic killer. It has destroyed my family and it will continue to take our loved ones away until we can educate people. Some time ago, we received the following e-mail from Erin's genetic counselor. It's comforting to know that our experience has already begun something of a chain reaction of information and education:

"*Your family has done such a tremendous job in getting the word out about this disease. We have received phone calls from numerous provinces, requesting information for relatives who have come forward for testing. Our number of referrals from doctors asking about this condition has also increased dramatically since we met with your family. Erin truly has left behind a legacy that has provided countless people with a way to take charge of their own health. You're doing the best you can, and know that we will always be here when people are ready."*

Appendix C
CHOICES

Today we have the opportunity to make a choice when it comes to planning a family. In the wake of discovering that Erin's cousin Summer had tested positive for the CDH1 mutation while pregnant, it becomes important to know what options are available for high-risk individuals who want children. In vitro fertilization was introduced to offer couples having trouble with conception. According to Wikipedia, in Vitro names "a process by which egg cells are fertilized by sperm outside the womb."[10] Medical support can be provided in planning the pregnancy, and doctors can now offer individuals with specific genetic mutations

In Vitro Fertilization with Preimplantation Genetic Screening (PDS)

This is useful to identify if the pregnancy is normal or abnormal, e.g. carrying a mutation. A method widely used in in vitro is what is known as "Intracytoplasmic Sperm Injection" (ICSI).

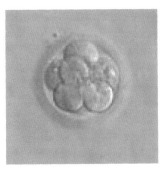

"Naked" Egg 8-Cell embryo 72 hrs after fertilization

10 Wikipedia: http://en.wikipedia.org/wiki/In_vitro_fertilisation. Accessed June 1, 2014.

Another method used in conception is placing sperm into a dish close to the egg, but it has to penetrate the egg on its own. "Confirmed figures are hard to come by, but it is estimated that since 1984–2008 (350,000 to 1/2 million IVF babies have been born)."[11]

I was able to find two locations in Canada that offer Genetic Screening PGD, located in Calgary and Montreal. See the website for the McGill University Reproductive Centre for more information.[12]

According to Katherine at Young Adult Cancer, "Generally, people would need to get a referral through a reproductive specialist for one of these clinics. If someone wanted to pursue this, they should ask their physician or genetic counselor how to get started."[13]

At the time of writing this book (2014), it depends on which Canadian province or territory you reside in. Each couple is a unique case with unique circumstances. Talk to a genetic counselor and inquire about Preimplantation Genetic Screening; some of these services might be covered by Canadian Medicare. If not, the estimated cost of PGD testing is steep: around $10.000.

Genesis Genetics does the majority of PGD testing in the United States and lists CDH1 as one of the genetic mutations they screen.[14]

11 Wikipedia: http://en.wikipedia.org/wiki/In_vitro_fertilisation) Accessed June 1, 2014.
12 McGill University Reproductive Centre: www.mcgillivf.com/e/McgillIVF.asp Accessed June 1, 2014.
13 www.YoungAdultCancer.ca. Access June 1, 2014.
14 Genesis Genetics: http://genesisgenetics.org/pgd/what-we-test-for/. Accessed June 1, 2014.

Printed in Canada